Big Data in Dental Research and Oral Healthcare

Big Data in Dental Research and Oral Healthcare

Editor

Tim Joda

MDPI • Basel • Beijing • Wuhan • Barcelona • Belgrade • Manchester • Tokyo • Cluj • Tianjin

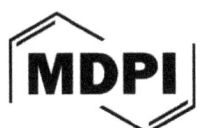

Editor
Tim Joda
University of Basel
Switzerland

Editorial Office
MDPI
St. Alban-Anlage 66
4052 Basel, Switzerland

This is a reprint of articles from the Special Issue published online in the open access journal *International Journal of Environmental Research and Public Health* (ISSN 1660-4601) (available at: https://www.mdpi.com/journal/ijerph/special_issues/BDIDR).

For citation purposes, cite each article independently as indicated on the article page online and as indicated below:

LastName, A.A.; LastName, B.B.; LastName, C.C. Article Title. *Journal Name* **Year**, *Volume Number*, Page Range.

ISBN 978-3-0365-0456-8 (Hbk)
ISBN 978-3-0365-0457-5 (PDF)

© 2021 by the authors. Articles in this book are Open Access and distributed under the Creative Commons Attribution (CC BY) license, which allows users to download, copy and build upon published articles, as long as the author and publisher are properly credited, which ensures maximum dissemination and a wider impact of our publications.

The book as a whole is distributed by MDPI under the terms and conditions of the Creative Commons license CC BY-NC-ND.

Contents

About the Editor . . . . **vii**

Preface to "Big Data in Dental Research and Oral Healthcare" . . . . **ix**

Tim Joda, Michael M. Bornstein, Ronald E. Jung, Marco Ferrari, Tuomas Waltimo and Nicola U. Zitzmann
Recent Trends and Future Direction of Dental Research in the Digital Era
Reprinted from: *Int. J. Environ. Res. Public Health* **2020**, *17*, 1987, doi:10.3390/ijerph17061987 . . . **1**

Christian E. Besimo, Nicola U. Zitzmann and Tim Joda
Digital Oral Medicine for the Elderly
Reprinted from: *Int. J. Environ. Res. Public Health* **2020**, *17*, 2171, doi:10.3390/ijerph17072171 . . **9**

Nicola U. Zitzmann, Lea Matthisson, Harald Ohla and Tim Joda
Digital Undergraduate Education in Dentistry: A Systematic Review
Reprinted from: *Int. J. Environ. Res. Public Health* **2020**, *17*, 3269, doi:10.3390/ijerph17093269 . . . **15**

Sung Eun Choi, Lisa Simon, Jane R. Barrow, Nathan Palmer, Sanjay Basu and Russell S. Phillips
Dental Practice Integration Into Primary Care: A Microsimulation of Financial Implications for Practices
Reprinted from: *Int. J. Environ. Res. Public Health* **2020**, *17*, 2154, doi:10.3390/ijerph17062154 . . **39**

Kuofeng Hung, Andy Wai Kan Yeung, Ray Tanaka and Michael M. Bornstein
Current Applications, Opportunities, and Limitations of AI for 3D Imaging in Dental Research and Practice
Reprinted from: *Int. J. Environ. Res. Public Health* **2020**, *17*, 4424, doi:10.3390/ijerph17124424 . . **53**

Yoshiaki Nomura, Yoshimasa Ishii, Yota Chiba, Shunsuke Suzuki, Akira Suzuki, Senichi Suzuki, Kenji Morita, Joji Tanabe, Koji Yamakawa, Yasuo Ishiwata, Meu Ishikawa, Kaoru Sogabe, Erika Kakuta, Ayako Okada, Ryoko Otsuka and Nobuhiro Hanada
Does Last Year's Cost Predict the Present Cost? An Application of Machine Leaning for the Japanese Area-Basis Public Health Insurance Database
Reprinted from: *Int. J. Environ. Res. Public Health* **2021**, *18*, 565, doi:10.3390/ijerph18020565 . . . **71**

Maddalena Favaretto, David Shaw, Eva De Clercq, Tim Joda and Bernice Simone Elger
Big Data and Digitalization in Dentistry: A Systematic Review of the Ethical Issues
Reprinted from: *Int. J. Environ. Res. Public Health* **2020**, *17*, 2495, doi:10.3390/ijerph17072495 . . . **85**

About the Editor

Tim Joda is the Vice Chair, Head of Dental Technology & Digital Dental Solutions, and Director of the Postgraduate Education Program at the Department of Reconstructive Dentistry, of the University Center for Dental Medicine Basel, Switzerland. He is the principle investigator and actively participates in clinical and translational research related to implant workflows and prosthetic treatment concepts in the field of digital dental technologies and e-health data management using AI and ML.

Preface to "Big Data in Dental Research and Oral Healthcare"

Digital transformation is a game changer in the present era, and digitalization in oral healthcare is recognized as the key promoter for evidence-based dentistry, improving diagnostics, prevention and therapy protocols. The future direction of dental medicine aims to close the gap between oral and general health by considering patient-centered outcomes and personalized medicine to secure patients' quality of life. Nevertheless, different data sources and formats without uniform standards and uncertainty related to patient security and privacy inhibit the ubiquitous use of health data to generate medical- and social-added value.

In general, the core requirements for clinical research to be efficient, successful, and competitive comprise the establishment of adequate infrastructure, as well as the coordination and harmonization of data flows, including well-trained experts in the interest of society. With the explosion of generated health data, dental medicine is edging into its next stage of digitization using big data and AI technology. Today, the dental profession is facing new challenges for clinical routine work. The most valuable area of interest for AI/ML is diagnostic imaging in dento-maxillofacial radiology for the identification of landmarks, oral pathologies, and automatically generated dental records. In this context, electronic health records are the mandatory door opener to personalized medicine. Moreover, the linkage of patient-level information to population-based citizen cohorts and biobanks provides the required reference of diagnostic and screening cutoffs that could identify new biomarkers and develop predictive models through personalized health research.

In addition to technically oriented applications in diagnostics and patient therapy, digitalization will revolutionarily influence the entire field of under- and postgraduate dental education, e.g., e-learning platforms facilitating 24/7 access and simulated motorskill training using AR/VR technology. Recently, COVID-19 has shown that virtual classrooms are a serious alternative to traditional in-person teaching. Digitalization will also have a major impact in helping deal with the complex challenges in oral medicine for the growing elderly population.

Digitally optimized operations ensure the efficient utilization of value-based healthcare services with seamless patient experience promoting health economics with balanced costs. However, digital technologies are not available everywhere. There is a growing realization that integrating dental and primary care may provide comprehensive care.

Finally, digitalization is raising novel and unpredictable challenges in the biomedical context. Ethical issues related to big data in terms of the systematic collection, sharing, and analysis of patient-specific health data must be discussed and solved considering all stakeholders, such as patients, healthcare providers, university and research institutions, medtech industry, insurance, public media, and state policy.

Tim Joda
Editor

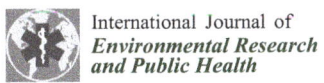

International Journal of
Environmental Research and Public Health

Letter

Recent Trends and Future Direction of Dental Research in the Digital Era

Tim Joda [1,*], Michael M. Bornstein [2], Ronald E. Jung [3], Marco Ferrari [4], Tuomas Waltimo [2] and Nicola U. Zitzmann [1]

1. Department of Reconstructive Dentistry, University Center for Dental Medicine Basel, University of Basel, 4058 Basel, Switzerland; n.zitzmann@unibas.ch
2. Department of Oral Health & Medicine, University Center for Dental Medicine Basel, University of Basel, 4058 Basel, Switzerland; michael.bornstein@unibas.ch (M.M.B.); tuomas.waltimo@unibas.ch (T.W.)
3. Department of Reconstructive Dentistry, Center for Dental Medicine Basel, University of Zurich, 8032 Zurich, Switzerland; ronald.jung@zzm.uzh.ch
4. Department of Prosthodontics & Dental Material, University School of Dental Medicine, University of Siena, 53100 Siena, Italy; ferrarm@gmail.com
* Correspondence: tim.joda@unibas.ch; Tel.: +41-61-267-2630

Received: 4 March 2020; Accepted: 10 March 2020; Published: 18 March 2020

Abstract: The digital transformation in dental medicine, based on electronic health data information, is recognized as one of the major game-changers of the 21st century to tackle present and upcoming challenges in dental and oral healthcare. This opinion letter focuses on the estimated top five trends and innovations of this new digital era, with potential to decisively influence the direction of dental research: (1) rapid prototyping (RP), (2) augmented and virtual reality (AR/VR), (3) artificial intelligence (AI) and machine learning (ML), (4) personalized (dental) medicine, and (5) tele-healthcare. Digital dentistry requires managing expectations pragmatically and ensuring transparency for all stakeholders: patients, healthcare providers, university and research institutions, the medtech industry, insurance, public media, and state policy. It should not be claimed or implied that digital smart data technologies will replace humans providing dental expertise and the capacity for patient empathy. The dental team that controls digital applications remains the key and will continue to play the central role in treating patients. In this context, the latest trend word is created: augmented intelligence, e.g., the meaningful combination of digital applications paired with human qualities and abilities in order to achieve improved dental and oral healthcare, ensuring quality of life.

Keywords: digital transformation; rapid prototyping; augmented and virtual reality (AR/VR); artificial intelligence (AI); machine learning (ML); personalized dental medicine; tele-health; patient-centered outcomes

---

1. Introduction

Digital transformation is the ubiquitous catchword in a variety of business sectors, and (dental) medicine is no exception [1]. Continuous progress in information technology (IT) has made it possible to overcome the limitations and hurdles that existed in clinical and technological workflows just a few years ago [2]. In addition, social and cultural behaviors of civilized society in industrial countries have changed and fostered the trend of digitalization: urbanism, centralization, and mobility, permanent accessibility via smartphones and tablets combined with the internet of things (IoT), as well as convenience-driven markets striving for efficiency [3].

The implementation of digital tools and applications reveals novel options facing today's chief problems in healthcare, such as a demographic development of an aging population with an increased prevalence of chronic diseases and increased treatment costs over an individual's lifespan [4]. In dental medicine, several digital workflows for production processing have already been integrated into treatment protocols, especially in the rapidly growing branch of computer-aided design/computer-aided manufacturing (CAD/CAM) and rapid prototyping (RP) [5].

New possibilities have opened up for automated processing in radiological imaging using artificial intelligence (AI) and machine learning (ML). Moreover, augmented and virtual reality (AR/VR) is the technological basis for the superimposition of diverse imaging files creating virtual dental patients and non-invasive simulations comparing different outcomes prior to any clinical intervention. Increased IT-power has fostered these promising technologies, whose possible uses can only be assessed in the future [6]. Not all digital options are currently exhausted, and their (valuable) advantages are not completely understood. Basic science, clinical trials, and subsequently derived knowledge for innovative therapy protocols need to be re-directed towards patient-centered outcomes, enabling the linkage of oral and general health instead of merely industry-oriented investigations [7].

To sum up, unseen opportunities will arise due to digital transformation in oral healthcare and dental research. Therefore, this opinion letter highlights the estimated top five healthcare trends and innovations of the dawning digital era that might influence the direction of dental research and their stakeholders in the near future.

2. Top Five Healthcare Trends and Innovations

2.1. Rapid Prototyping (RP)

RP is a technique to quickly and automatically construct three-dimensional (3D) models of a final product or a part of a whole using 3D-printers. The additive manufacturing process allows inexpensive production of complex 3D-geometries from various materials and minimal material wastage [8]. However, while the future looks very promising from a technical and scientific point of view, it is not clear how RP and its products will be regulated. This uncertainty is problematic for the producing industry, healthcare provider, and patients as well.

In dentistry, one of the main difficulties today is the choice of materials. Commercially available materials commonly used for RP are currently permitted for short to medium-term intraoral retention only and are, therefore, limited to temporary restorations and not yet intended for definitive dental reconstructions. RP offers great potential in dental technology for mass production of dental models, but also for the fabrication of implant surgical guides [9]. For those indications, prolonged intraoral retention is not required. From an economic point of view, a great advantage is the production in large quantities at the same time in a reproducible and standardized way. Another important area of application is the use of 3D-printed models in dental education based on CBCT or μCT. An initial study, however, has revealed that 3D-printed dental models can show changes in dimensional accuracy over periods of 4 weeks and longer. In this context, further investigations comparing different 3D-printers and material combinations are compellingly necessary for clarification [10].

In the near future, those material-related barriers and limitations will probably be broken down. Many research groups are focusing on the development of printable materials for dental reconstructions, such as zirconium dioxide (ZrO_2) [11]. This different mode of fabrication of ZrO_2 structures could allow us to realize totally innovative geometries with hollow bodies that might be used, for example, for time-dependent low-dose release of anti-inflammatory agents in implant dentistry [12]. A completely revolutionary aspect would be the synthesis of biomaterials to artificially create lost tooth structures using RP technology [13]. Instead of using a preformed dental tooth databank, a patient-specific digital dental dataset could be acquired at the time of growth completion and used for future dental reconstructions. Furthermore, the entire tooth can be duplicated to serve as an individualized implant. RP will most likely offer low-cost production and highly customized solutions in various fields of dental medicine that can be tailored to suit the specific needs of each patient.

2.2. Augmented and Virtual Reality (AR/VR)

AR is an interactive technology enhancing a real-world environment by computer-animated perceptual information. In other words, AR expands the real world with virtual content. In most cases, it is the superimposition of additional digital information on live images or videos. VR, in contrast, uses only artificial computerized scenarios without connection to reality [14]. Depending on the technique, every conceivable way of sensation can be used, mainly visual, auditory, and haptic, independently or in any combination [15]. Today, there is a rapidly increasing number of applications for AR/VR technologies in dental medicine as a whole, as well as many intriguing developments for both patients and healthcare providers [16–18].

AR/VR software allows users to superimpose virtually created visualizations onto recordings of the patient in natural motion. Any 3D-model, for instance, a prosthetic design of a possible reconstruction, can be augmented into the individual patient situation to simulate diverse, prospective outcomes in advance without invasive work steps [19]. These digital models can then be viewed in real-time and facilitate communication not only with the patient to demystify the complex treatment steps but also between dental professionals to make the treatment more predictable and efficient. In the future, the possibilities will continue to grow and help facilitate the dental routine. An interesting indication is the augmentation of CBCT-based virtual implant planning directly into the oral cavity or while using intraoral scanners (IOS), projection, and display of the optically detected area with AR glasses.

Another promising area of interest is the sector of dental education, transferring theoretical knowledge and practical exercises to offer interactive teaching with 24/7-access and objective evaluation. AR/VR-based motor skill training for tooth preparation especially facilitates efficient and autonomous learning for dental students. Initial studies have shown that AR/VR technologies stimulate more senses to learn meritoriously [20]. Moreover, in postgraduate education, challenging and complex clinical protocols can be trained in a complete virtual environment without risk or harm for real patients; additionally, specialists can continuously maintain their skills while training with AR/VR-simulations. Within a few years, AR/VR will have the potential to revolutionize dental education radically [21,22].

2.3. Artificial Intelligence (AI) and Machine Learning (ML)

AI (including ML) has already invaded and established itself in our daily lives, although in more subtle means, such as virtual assistants named "Siri" or "Alexa". The basis for AI is the increasing power of computers to think like and complete tasks currently performed by humans with greater speed, accuracy, and lower resource utilization [23,24]. Therefore, AI technology is perfect for work that requires the analysis and evaluation of large amounts of data. Repetitive activities are boring and tiring for humans in the long-run with increased risk of error, while AI-based applications do not show signs of fatigue. In contrast to humans, the artificial learning process results in constant better performance with increasing workload. Additionally, computers are not biased compared to humans, who come with innate biases and may judge things prematurely and differently from each other [25,26].

The most valuable indication for the use of AI and ML in dentistry is the entire field of diagnostic imaging in dento-maxillofacial radiology [27,28]. Currently, applications and research in AI purposes in dental radiology focus on automated localization of cephalometric landmarks, diagnosis of osteoporosis, classification/segmentation of maxillofacial cysts and/or tumors, and identification of periodontitis/periapical disease. Computer software analyzing radiographs has to be trained on huge datasets ("big data") to recognize meaningful patterns. The diagnostic performance of AI models varies among different algorithms used, is also dependent on the observers labeling the datasets, and it is still necessary to verify the generalizability and reliability of these models by using adequate, representative images. AI software must be able to understand new information presented by images as well as written text or spoken language with proper context. Finally, the software must be able to make intelligent decisions regarding this new information, and then, learn from mistakes to improve the decision-making for future processing [29].

A beneficial AI system should realize all of this in about the same time that a human being can perform the given task. Up to now, applications of AI on a broad scale were not technically feasible or cost-effective, so the reality of AI has not yet matched the possibilities in routine dental applications [30], although the technical progress is exponential, and very soon, a large number of AI models will be developed for automated diagnostics of 3D-imaging identifying pathologies, prediction of disease risk, to propose potential therapeutic options, and to evaluate prognosis.

2.4. Personalized (Dental) Medicine

Electronic health records (eHR) with standardized diagnostics and generally accepted data formats are the mandatory door opener to personalized medicine and predictive models investigating a broader population. The structured assessment and systematic collection of patient information is an effective instrument in health economics [31]. Health data can be obtained from routine dental healthcare and clinical trials, as well as from diverse new sources, as IoT in general, and specifically, data on the social determinants of health [3].

The linkage of individual patient data gathered from various sources enables the diagnosis of rare diseases and completely novel strategies for research [32]. Examining large population-based patient cohorts could detect unidentified correlations of diseases and create prognostic models for new treatment concepts. The linkage of patient-level information to population-based citizen cohorts and biobanks provides the required reference of diagnostic and screening cutoffs that could identify new biomarkers through personalized health research [33].

eHR has great power for a change of research both ways. On the other side, the digitized transparent patient could be stigmatized and categorized by insurance companies, provoking adverse effects that have not yet been determined socially [3,6]. Therefore, linked biomedical data supporting register-based research pose several risks and methodological challenges for clinical research: appropriate security settings and the development of algorithms for statistical calculations, including interpretation of collected health data [34,35]. A generally accepted code of conduct has to be defined and established for the ethical and meaningful use of register-based patient data.

Overall, personalized medicine holds the key to unlocking a new frontier in dental research. Genomic sequencing, combined with the developments in medical imaging and regenerative technology, has redefined personalized medicine using novel molecular tools to perform patient-specific precision healthcare [36,37]. It has the potential to revolutionize healthcare using genomics information for individual biomarker identification [38]. The vision is an interdisciplinary approach to dental patient sample analysis, in which dentists, physicians, and nurses can collaborate to understand the inter-connectivity of disease in a cost-effective way [39].

2.5. Tele-Healthcare

Tele-healthcare enables a convenient way for patients to increase self-care while potentially reducing office visits and travel time [40]. Considering the growing number of the elderly population with reduced mobility and/or nursing home-stay, special-care patients, as well as people living in rural areas, these patient groups would benefit significantly from tele-dentistry [41,42]. Measures to be taken in case of dental trauma can be effectively communicated by telephone counselors and can be frequently used during out-of-office hours [43]. In general, it facilitates easier access to care and also represents a cost-reduced option for patients, as instead of expensive treatments, tele-dentistry shifts towards prevention practices and allows patients to consult with otherwise unavailable dental professionals, for example, using a live consult via video-streaming [44,45]. Nevertheless, it must be emphasized that tele-dentistry can never replace a real dentist; rather, it must be understood as an additional tool [30].

Today, tele-dentistry is only in an early start-up phase [46]. Early studies have mainly focused on specific and rare diseases that might require surgery, but there are findings that suggest that a teleradiology system in general dental practice could be helpful for the differential diagnosis of common lesions and may result in a reduction of unnecessary costs [47]. There is a fundamental need to regulate the expanding field of tele-healthcare, with guidelines to secure clinical quality standards. The legislation must be clearly defined and clarified for routine implementation of a national-wide tele-dentistry platform. The technical requirements must be met and security standards for sensitive patient information guaranteed, with well-defined regulatory affairs.

3. Conclusions

The future direction of dental research should foster the linkage of oral and general health in order to focus on personalized medicine considering patient-centered outcomes. In this context, dental research must have an impact as a deliverable to society, not just research to churn out scientific publications but to truly change protocols applied in the clinic. Moreover, here, digitization with AI/ML and AR/VR represents the most promising tools for innovative research today. Furthermore, research in a digital era will also be more and more assessed in terms of "impact" as a deliverable good. Impact assessment is still very much debated by scientists, healthcare policy-makers, and politicians. Additionally, general public health societies are increasingly dependent on solid data sets, gaining knowledge to enable innovations and result in recommendations, guidelines, and healthcare policies of utmost importance. These are supposed to generate economic and social benefits on every and each level from an individual to a population. Scientists in dental medicine have also to be aware that funding might be increasingly dependent on the possibility to demonstrate an impact on a large scale. Thus, the use of impact assessments in the future will most likely serve the following two tasks: (1) demonstrating the value of research, and (2) increasing the value of research through a more effective way of financing research in order to have a societal impact [48,49].

For digital dentistry, this requires managing expectations pragmatically and ensuring transparency for all stakeholders: patients, healthcare providers, university and other research institutions, the medtech industry, insurance, public media, and state policy. It should not be claimed or implied that digital smart data technologies will replace humans who possess dental expertise and the capacity for patient empathy. Therefore, the dental team controlling the power of the digital toolbox is the key and will continue to play a central role in the patient's journey to receive the best possible individual treatment, and to provide emotional support. The collection, storage, and analysis of digitized biomedical patient data pose several challenges. In addition to technical aspects for the handling of huge amounts of data, considering internationally defined standards, an ethical and meaningful policy must ensure the protection of patient data for safety optimal impact.

Nowadays, the mixed term "augmented intelligence" is perhaps somewhat prematurely introduced in social media. However, the benefits of digital applications will complement human qualities and abilities in order to achieve improved and cost-efficient healthcare for patients. Augmented intelligence based on big data will help to reduce the incidence of misdiagnosis and offers more useful insights—quickly, accurately, and easily. This is all achievable without losing the human touch, improving the quality of life.

Author Contributions: Conceptualization, T.J.; Methodology, T.J. and N.U.Z.; Writing—Original Draft Preparation, T.J. and N.U.Z.; Writing—Review and Editing, M.M.B., R.E.J., M.F., and T.W.; Supervision, T.J.; Project Administration, T.J. All authors have read and agreed to the published version of the manuscript.

Funding: This research received no external funding.

Conflicts of Interest: The authors declare no conflict of interest.

References

1. Gopal, G.; Suter-Crazzolara, C.; Toldo, L. Digital transformation in healthcare—Architectures of present and future information technologies. *Clin. Chem. Lab. Med.* **2019**, *57*, 328–335. [CrossRef] [PubMed]
2. Weber, G.M.; Mandl, K.D.; Kohane, I.S. Finding the missing link for big biomedical data. *J. Am. Med. Assoc.* **2014**, *311*, 2479–2480. [CrossRef] [PubMed]

3. Joda, T.; Waltimo, T.; Pauli-Magnus, C.; Probst-Hensch, N.; Zitzmann, N.U. Population-based linkage of big data in dental research. *Int. J. Environ. Res. Public Health* **2018**, *15*, 2357. [CrossRef] [PubMed]
4. Glick, M. Taking a byte out of big data. *J. Am. Dent. Assoc.* **2015**, *146*, 793–794. [CrossRef]
5. Miyazaki, T.; Hotta, Y. CAD/CAM systems available for the fabrication of crown and bridge restorations. *Aust. Dent. J.* **2011**, *56* (Suppl. 1), 97–106. [CrossRef]
6. Jones, K.H.; Laurie, G.; Stevens, L.; Dobbs, C.; Ford, D.V.; Lea, N. The other side of the coin: Harm due to the non-use of health-related data. *Int. J. Med. Inform.* **2017**, *97*, 43–51. [CrossRef]
7. Joda, T.; Waltimo, T.; Probst-Hensch, N.; Pauli-Magnus, C.; Zitzmann, N.U. Health data in dentistry: An attempt to master the digital challenge. *Public Health Genom.* **2019**, *22*, 1–7. [CrossRef]
8. Joda, T.; Ferrari, M.; Gallucci, G.O.; Wittenben, J.-G.; Bragger, U. Digital technology in fixed implant prosthodontics. *Periodontology 2000* **2017**, *73*, 178–192. [CrossRef]
9. Dawood, A.; Marti Marti, B.; Sauret-Jackson, V.; Darwood, A. 3D printing in dentistry. *Br. Dent. J.* **2015**, *219*, 521–529. [CrossRef]
10. Lech, G.; Nordström, E. Dimensional Stability of 3D Printed Dental Models. Master's Thesis, Malmö University Electronic Publishing, Malmö, Sweden, 2018.
11. Galantea, R.; Figueiredo-Pinaa, C.G.; Serro, A.P. Additive manufacturing of ceramics for dental applications: A review. *Dent. Mater.* **2019**, *35*, 825–846. [CrossRef]
12. Zocca, A.; Colombo, P.; Gomes, C.M.; Gunster, J. Additive manufacturing of ceramics: Issues, potentialities, and opportunities. *J. Am. Ceram. Soc.* **2015**, *98*, 1983–2001. [CrossRef]
13. Bose, S.; Ke, D.; Sahasrabudhe, H.; Bandyopadhyay, A. Additive manufacturing of biomaterials. *Prog. Mater. Sci.* **2018**, *93*, 45–111. [CrossRef] [PubMed]
14. Sutherland, J.; Belec, J.; Sheikh, A.; Chepelev, L.; Althobaity, W.; Chow, B.J.W.; Mitsouras, D.; Christensen, A.; Rybicki, F.J.; La Russa, D.J. Applying modern virtual and augmented reality technologies to medical images and models. *J. Digit. Imaging* **2019**, *32*, 38–53. [CrossRef] [PubMed]
15. Pensieri, C.; Pennacchini, M. Overview: Virtual reality in medicine. *J. Virtual Worlds Res.* **2014**, *7*, 1–34. [CrossRef]
16. Kwon, H.B.; Park, Y.S.; Han, J.S. Augmented reality in dentistry: A current perspective. *Acta Odontol. Scand.* **2018**, *76*, 497–503. [CrossRef]
17. Joda, T.; Gallucci, G.O.; Wismeijer, D.; Zitzmann, N.U. Augmented and virtual reality in dental medicine: A systematic review. *Comput. Biol. Med.* **2019**, *108*, 93–100. [CrossRef]
18. Farronato, M.; Maspero, C.; Lanteri, V.; Fama, A.; Ferrati, F.; Pettenuzzo, A.; Farronato, D. Current state of the art in the use of augmented reality in dentistry: A systematic review of the literature. *BMC Oral Health* **2019**, *19*, 135. [CrossRef]
19. Joda, T.; Gallucci, G.O. The virtual patient in dental medicine. *Clin. Oral Implant. Res.* **2015**, *26*, 725–726. [CrossRef]
20. Lee, S.H. Research and development of haptic simulator for dental education using virtual reality and user motion. *Int. J. Adv. Smart Conv.* **2018**, *7*, 114–120.
21. Ayoub, A.; Pulijala, Y. The application of virtual reality and augmented reality in Oral & Maxillofacial Surgery. *BMC Oral Health* **2019**, *19*, 238.
22. Durham, M.; Engel, B.; Ferrill, T.; Halford, J.; Singh, T.P.; Gladwell, M. Digitally augmented learning in implant dentistry. *Oral Maxillofac. Surg. Clin. N. Am.* **2019**, *31*, 387–398. [CrossRef] [PubMed]
23. Currie, G. Intelligent imaging: Anatomy of machine learning and deep learning. *J. Nucl. Med. Technol.* **2019**, *47*, 273–281. [CrossRef] [PubMed]
24. Park, W.J.; Park, J.B. History and application of artificial neural networks in dentistry. *Eur. J. Dent.* **2018**, *12*, 594–601. [CrossRef] [PubMed]
25. Chen, Y.W.; Stanley, K.; Att, W. Artificial intelligence in dentistry: Current applications and future perspectives. *Quintessence Int.* **2020**, *51*, 248–257. [PubMed]
26. Kulkarni, S.; Seneviratne, N.; Baig, M.S.; Khan, A.H.A. Artificial intelligence in medicine: Where are we now? *Acad. Radiol.* **2020**, *27*, 62–70. [CrossRef] [PubMed]
27. Tuzoff, D.V.; Tuzova, L.N.; Bornstein, M.M.; Krasnov, A.S.; Kharchenko, M.A.; Nikolenko, S.I.; Sveshnikov, M.M.; Bednenko, G.B. Tooth detection and numbering in panoramic radiographs using convolutional neural networks. *Dentomaxillofac. Radiol.* **2019**, *48*, 20180051. [CrossRef]

28. Hung, K.; Montalvao, C.; Tanaka, R.; Kawai, T.; Bornstein, M.M. The use and performance of artificial intelligence applications in dental and maxillofacial radiology: A systematic review. *Dentomaxillofac. Radiol.* **2020**, *49*, 20190107. [CrossRef]
29. Leite, A.F.; Vasconcelos, K.F.; Willems, H.; Jacobs, R. Radiomics and machine learning in oral healthcare. *Proteom. Clin. Appl.* **2020**, e1900040, [Epub ahead of print]. [CrossRef]
30. Goldhahn, J.; Rampton-Branco-Weiss, V.; Spinas, G.A. Could artificial intelligence make doctors obsolete? *BMJ* **2018**, *363*, k4563. [CrossRef] [PubMed]
31. Tokede, O.; White, J.; Stark, P.C.; Vaderhobli, R.; Walji, M.F.; Ramoni, R.; Schoonheim-Klein, M.; Kimmes, N.; Tavares, A.; Kalenderian, E. Assessing use of a standardized dental diagnostic terminology in an electronic health record. *J. Dent. Educ.* **2013**, *77*, 24–36. [PubMed]
32. Harron, K.L.; Doidge, J.C.; Knight, H.E.; Gilbert, R.E.; Goldstein, H.; Cromwell, D.A.; van der Meulen, J.H. A guide to evaluating linkage quality for the analysis of linked data. *Int. J. Epidemiol.* **2017**, *46*, 1699–1710. [CrossRef] [PubMed]
33. Manolopoulos, V.G.; Dechairo, B.; Huriez, A.; Kühn, A.; Llerena, A.; van Schaik, R.H.; Yeo, K.T.; Ragia, G.; Siest, G. Pharmacogenomics and personalized medicine in clinical practice. *Pharmacogenomics* **2011**, *12*, 597–610. [CrossRef] [PubMed]
34. Aldridge, R.W.; Shaji, K.; Hayward, A.C.; Abubakar, I. Accuracy of probabilistic linkage using the enhanced matching system for public health and epidemiological studies. *PLoS ONE* **2015**, *10*, e0136179. [CrossRef] [PubMed]
35. Jorm, L. Routinely collected data as a strategic resource for research: Priorities for methods and workforce. *Public Health Res. Pract.* **2015**, *25*, e2541540. [CrossRef]
36. Garcia, I.; Kuska, R.; Somerman, M.J. Expanding the foundation for personalized medicine: Implications and challenges for dentistry. *J. Dent. Res.* **2013**, *92*, 3–10. [CrossRef]
37. Marrazzo, P.; Paduano, F.; Palmieri, F.; Marrelli, M.; Tatullo, M. Highly efficient in vitro reparative behavior of dental pulp stem cells cultured with standardized platelet lysate. *Stem Cells Int.* **2016**, *2016*, 7230987. [CrossRef]
38. Emmert-Streib, F. Personalized medicine: Has it started yet? A reconstruction of the early history. *Front. Genet.* **2013**, *3*, 313. [CrossRef]
39. Di Sanzo, M.; Borro, M.; La Russa, R.; Cipolloni, L.; Santurro, A.; Scopetti, M.; Simmaco, M.; Frati, P. Clinical applications of personalized medicine: A new paradigm and challenge. *Curr. Pharm. Biotechnol.* **2017**, *18*, 194–203. [CrossRef]
40. Wang, S.; Parsons, M.; Stone-McLean, J.; Rogers, P.; Boyd, S.; Hoover, K.; Meruvis-Pastor, O.; Gong, M.; Smith, A. Augmented reality as a telemedicine platform for remote procedural training. *Sensors* **2017**, *17*, 2294. [CrossRef]
41. Jampani, N.D.; Nutalapati, R.; Dontula, B.S.; Boyapati, R. Applications of teledentistry: A literature review and update. *J. Int. Soc. Prev. Community Dent.* **2011**, *1*, 37–44.
42. Estai, M.; Kruger, E.; Tennant, M.; Bunt, S.; Kanagasingam, Y. Challenges in the uptake of telemedicine in dentistry. *Rural. Remote. Health* **2016**, *16*, 3915. [PubMed]
43. Lienert, N.; Zitzmann, N.U.; Filippi, A.; Weiger, R.; Krastl, G. Teledental consultations related to trauma in a Swiss telemedical center: A retrospective survey. *Dent. Traumatol.* **2010**, *26*, 223–227. [CrossRef] [PubMed]
44. Daniel, S.J.; Kumar, S. Teledentistry: A key component in access to care. *J. Evid. Based Dent. Pract.* **2014**, *14*, 201–208. [CrossRef] [PubMed]
45. Irving, M.; Stewart, R.; Spallek, H.; Blinkhom, A. Using teledentistry in clinical practice as an enabler to improve access to clinical care: A qualitative systematic review. *J. Telemed. Telecare* **2018**, *24*, 129–146. [CrossRef] [PubMed]
46. Wang, G.; Xiang, W.; Pickering, M. A cross-platform solution for light field based 3D telemedicine. *Comput. Methods Programs Biomed.* **2016**, *125*, 103–116. [CrossRef]
47. Estai, M.; Bunt, S.; Kanagasingam, Y.; Tennant, M. Cost savings from a teledentistry model for school dental screening: An Australian health system perspective. *Aust. Health Rev.* **2018**, *42*, 482–490. [CrossRef]

48. Greenhalgh, T.; Raftery, J.; Hanney, S.; Glover, M. Research impact: A narrative review. *BMC Med.* **2016**, *14*, 78. [CrossRef]
49. Newson, R.; King, L.; Rychetnik, L.; Milat, A.; Bauman, A. Looking both ways: A review of methods for assessing research impacts on policy and the policy utilisation of research. *Health Res. Policy Syst.* **2018**, *16*, 54. [CrossRef]

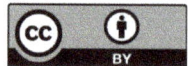

© 2020 by the authors. Licensee MDPI, Basel, Switzerland. This article is an open access article distributed under the terms and conditions of the Creative Commons Attribution (CC BY) license (http://creativecommons.org/licenses/by/4.0/).

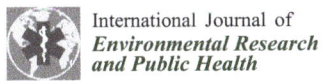

Letter

Digital Oral Medicine for the Elderly

Christian E. Besimo *, Nicola U. Zitzmann and Tim Joda

Department of Reconstructive Dentistry, University Center for Dental Medicine Basel, University of Basel, 4058 Basel, Switzerland; n.zitzmann@unibas.ch (N.U.Z.); tim.joda@unibas.ch (T.J.)
* Correspondence: christian.besimo@bluewin.ch; Tel.: +41-61-267-2632

Received: 16 February 2020; Accepted: 22 March 2020; Published: 25 March 2020

Abstract: Sustainable oral care of the elderly requires a holistic view of aging, which must extend far beyond the narrow field of dental expertise to help reduce the effects of sociobiological changes on oral health in good time. Digital technologies now extend into all aspects of daily life. This review summarizes the diverse digital opportunities that may help address the complex challenges in Gerodontology. Systemic patient management is at the center of these descriptions, while the application of digital tools for purely dental treatment protocols is deliberately avoided.

Keywords: oral medicine; oral healthcare; dentistry; gerodontology; elderly patient; digital transformation; big data; patient-centered outcomes

1. Introduction

The steady aging of human populations is a development that affects not only the industrialized world, but also emerging and developing countries. It is estimated that about half of all people who have ever lived to an age of 65 years old or older are alive today. We are living through an exponential population expansion and demographic transition. Therefore, it is necessary to understand the sociological and biological changes facing the elderly population and to master the current and future challenges in dental healthcare for aging patients [1].

This opinion letter, based on an ongoing evaluation of the sociodemographic changes due to aging, focuses on digital technologies, which could help deal with the complex challenges in oral medicine for the growing elderly.

2. A Silent Revolution

2.1. Social Change

Old age is changing fundamentally and to an extent that justifies the term 'social revolution', albeit one that is proceeding quietly. This change is characterized by the objective of being able to live in a self-determined manner and in a private environment for as long as possible, even when in need of healthcare. In this context, a transfer to a care institution is only foreseen in the case of an extreme emergency and to be delayed for as long as possible. This development will contribute to the progressive delaying of the fourth age, which is marked by the need for advanced assistance and care, and will further reduce the average length of stay in institutions. In Switzerland, individuals aged 65 years and older only stay in nursing homes for one year [2].

It is important to recognize the goal-oriented willingness and the high degree of creativity that senior citizens, either currently working or retired, display in their third age (traditionally 65–80 years old). However, these factors do not allow for any reliable prognoses regarding changes in lifestyles in old age and force the professional groups, institutions, and organizations concerned with aging to continually adapt their strategies and concepts [2]. This awareness has also reached the political arena in Switzerland, so that in future, there will be a growing reluctance to plan new inpatient care places and priority will be given to outpatient care in terms of cost-effectiveness [3,4].

2.2. Consequences for Health

The biological limit for life expectancy at birth and after reaching the age of 65 is still not predictable. Medical advances, healthy nutrition, good education, and improving working conditions continue to favor an increasingly longer third age and will reduce the risk and duration of the fourth age [2].

The preventive and restorative success of dentistry have led to people with an increasing number of teeth (including implant-supported reconstructions). However, despite their knowledge of the importance of regular dental check-ups for oral and general health, the elderly will inevitably gradually withdraw from this care, beginning between the ages of 60 and 65 [5]. The risk of psychosocial (loneliness, poverty) and medical problems (multimorbidity, polypharmacy), which increase with age, play a central role in withdrawing from care with major consequences for dental and oral health in the long term. Oral diseases do not only occur in old age when the need for help and care begins, but much earlier, because the social and biological factors mentioned above increasingly affect the resources needed to maintain oral hygiene and to receive regular care from the personal dental team. Even if the fourth age is delayed, the oral health issues still inevitably arise, and are then complicated further by the additional comorbidities of aging [6].

Facing these complex challenges, it is important for dentists to learn to perceive the human being holistically—in her or his entirety—and to establish a close network with other medical disciplines, institutions, organizations, authorities, and relatives who are concerned with the care of aging people. It is important to be aware that the range of stakeholders involved is growing and becoming more volatile, as the shift from inpatient to outpatient care increases [7,8].

3. Digital Opportunities

People participating in the digital community generate a rapidly growing amount of data every day. This is also increasingly true for senior citizens. Scientific use of this data offers the opportunity to gain a deeper and more dynamic insight into the lifestyle of aging people, for example, through analyzing digital shopping activities and payment transactions. This could allow a better and more up-to-date understanding of the changing lifestyles of the elderly. It is conceivable that algorithms could be developed that can identify sociobiological threats at an early stage by monitoring changes in behavior. Such algorithms would also be important for the dental care of aging people and thus for oral health. This would be one of several opportunities to achieve a paradigm shift in geriatric dentistry and to promote preventive rather than palliative care concepts that are still predominant [9,10].

3.1. In Frigo Veritas (The Truth Lies in the Fridge)

The *"In Frigo Veritas"* study conducted in Geneva in the 1990s demonstrated that the contents of the refrigerators of senior citizens was associated with the likelihood of hospitalization in the following month (11). Monitoring the nutritional provisions available to an elderly individual could therefore identify those at risk early. The use of shopping lists of food products, which are already electronically recorded today with the help of customer cards, could be considered here. This data alone would already allow individual conclusions to be drawn about the quantity, quality, and course of food. A link to intelligent refrigerator systems that can document the consumption and replenishment of food would also be conceivable. This would allow continuous conclusions to be drawn in real time on the nutritional situation and thus the morbidity risk in an out-of-home care setting [11]. This application could also be used in dentistry for therapeutic decision making or for the ongoing assessment of the care capacity of aging people threatened by sociobiological risks. In addition, nutritional counselling and guidance, supported by nutritional algorithms, could be carried out in a simplified, individualized and continuous manner, before, during, and/or after dental interventions such as tooth extractions or the insertion of fixed and removable dentures [12].

3.2. Intelligent, Individually Usable Systems

The personal health data generated in medicine, including dentistry, or by intelligent systems suitable for everyday use, such as smartphones, watches or other devices, open up a wide range of application options that will go far beyond the recording of acute emergency situations in in-home and out-of-home care settings. On the one hand, the cumulative use of medically relevant data does not only offer significantly expanded perspectives for research, but also for patient care. Today, it is already feasible to record vital data in real time using the aforementioned intelligent everyday systems. It can be assumed that the availability and variety of such systems will continuously increase in the near future and will also be usefully applied in dentistry [13,14].

3.3. Stop Walking When Talking

Nowadays, electronic pedometers are used to obtain discounts from health insurance companies. Similarly, we are already able to analyze gait regularity and thus the risk of falls among older people in specialized mobility centers, with or without multitasking, and to draw conclusions about diseases, side effects of medication, and cognitive performance [15]. The transfer of such systems to shoe insoles, for example, not only has the potential to obtain and link incomparably more empirical data on gait safety in elderly people living in a private household, but also to monitor their mobility in real time. In this context, the effects of therapeutic interventions on gait safety, such as those that aim to optimize occlusion, could be dynamically monitored [16].

4. Interdisciplinary Networking

As mentioned previously, the (dental) medical care of aging people living in private households is faced with growing interdisciplinary challenges. On the one hand, healthcare providers have to establish a network to harness the knowledge of the various disciplines by means of suitable digital systems to make it not only accessible for interdisciplinary research, but also clinically usable under growing organizational and legal requirements. On the other hand, everyday clinical practice requires dynamic, real-time networking among the growing number of stakeholders in the care of the elderly, which will increase significantly and become more volatile as outpatient care expands. Here, intelligent tools are needed that enable compatible, rapid, and secure interdisciplinary data exchange on a patient-by-patient basis to support individually tailored decision-making based on algorithms [17].

Finally, it is expected that routine sequencing of the genome in the case of disease will become established within the next five to ten years, as the costs of this procedure have been significantly reduced from $100,000 to $1000 over the last 20 years [18]. This should also contribute to the individualization of prevention, diagnostics, and therapy in dentistry, especially for older people with increasing psychosocial and medical risks. The latter could possibly be detected earlier and counteracted more effectively [19].

5. Ethical and Legal Responsibilities

We have learned from the hitherto short history of the digitalization of our world that this development is accelerating at a breathtaking rate. This calls for an urgent and internationally valid regulation for the protection of personal data of individuals, while enabling the exchange of personal information between stakeholders for the benefit of the individual. This has been pioneered by the basic data protection regulation of the European Union [20]. Such a set of rules must compensate for the existing socio-economic asymmetry of a data-driven economy, which ensures the right to a copy of personal data and thus digital self-determination. However, the right to a copy of personal data also requires the development of cooperatively managed databases that are able to manage the digital information in a fiduciary capacity and in a comparable way to financial institutions. In this way, it would be ensured that people could come into possession of all their health-related data to use these under regulated conditions for their own benefit or to make data available to research and thus to the community [21].

In addition, society must ensure that (dental) medicine, which is increasingly controlled by guidelines and algorithms, does not lose sight of the individual person. It is true that large amounts of data can increase the reliability of answers to individual questions. Nevertheless, it remains to be hoped that big data will not lead to further commercialization or industrialization of medicine, and thus, neglect the healing power of a systemic doctor-patient relationship, but rather that it will nurture this relationship [22,23].

6. Conclusions

The global demographic change is characterized by an exponential population expansion and sociobiological transition towards a growing number of older patients. Sustainable oral healthcare of the elderly must comprise a holistic view of aging, far beyond the narrow field of dental diagnostics and modernized treatment protocols. Digital health data generated in dental medicine, or by daily used systems, such as smartphones, tablets, and watches, open up a wide range of application options in (oral) healthcare to master the complex challenges in Gerodontology. Scientific use of this data offers broad insights into the lifestyle of aging patients for the early identification of social threats and changing behaviors.

Medical and dental healthcare providers have to establish an interdisciplinary network using these digital systems for routine clinical practice. Smart digital applications are needed, which enable compatible, rapid, and secure interdisciplinary data exchange on a patient-by-patient level to support individually tailored decision-making based on the knowledge of all stakeholders in the care of the elderly in in-home and out-of-home care settings. The digital transformation has the opportunity to achieve a paradigm shift in geriatric dentistry and to promote preventive rather than palliative healthcare concepts.

Author Contributions: Conceptualization, C.E.B. and T.J.; methodology, C.E.B. and T.J.; writing—original draft preparation, C.E.B.; writing—review and editing, T.J. and N.U.Z.; supervision, T.J.; project administration, T.J. All authors have read and agreed to the published version of the manuscript.

Funding: This research received no external funding.

Conflicts of Interest: The authors declare no conflicts of interest.

References

1. WHO. *World Report on Ageing and Health*; World Health Organization: Geneva, Switzerland, 2015.
2. Höpflinger, F.; Bayer-Oglesby, L.; Zumbrunn, A. *Pflegebedürftigkeit und Langzeitpflege im Alter. Aktualisierte Szenarien für die Schweiz*; Verlag Hans Huber: Bern, Switzerland, 2011; pp. 33–66.
3. Gesundheitsdirektion Kanton Zürich. *Bedarfsentwicklung und Steuerung der Stationären Pflegeplätze*; Kanton Zürich: Zürich, Switzerland, 2018.
4. Gesundheitsdepartement des Kantons Basel-Stadt. *Gesundheitsversorgungsbericht über die Spitäler, Pflegeheime, Tagespflegeheime und Spitex-Einrichtungen im Kanton Basel-Stadt*; Kanton Basel-Stadt: Basel, Switzerland, 2018.
5. Biffar, R.; Klinke-Wilberg, T. Gesundheit der Älterwerdenden und Inanspruchnahme ärztlicher Dienste—zahnmedizinische Konsequenzen und Aufgaben. *Senioren-Zahnmedizin* **2013**, *1*, 35–42.
6. Tavares, M.; Lindefjeld Calabi, K.A.; San Martin, L. Systemic diseases and oral health. *Dent. Clin. N. Am.* **2014**, *58*, 797–814. [CrossRef] [PubMed]
7. Plasschaert, A.J.M.; Holbrook, W.P.; Delap, E.; Martinez, C.; Walmsley, A.D. Profile and competences for the European dentist. *Eur. J. Dent. Educ.* **2005**, *9*, 98–107. [CrossRef] [PubMed]
8. Besimo, C. Paradigmenwechsel zugunsten einer besseren oralen Gesundheit im Alter. *Swiss Dent. J.* **2015**, *125*, 599–604. [PubMed]
9. March, S. Individual Data Linkage of Survey Data with Claims Data in Germany—An Overview Based on a Cohort Study. *Int. J. Environ. Res. Public Health* **2017**, *14*, 1543–1558. [CrossRef] [PubMed]

10. Joda, T.; Waltimo, T.; Pauli-Magnus, C.; Probst-Hensch, N.; Zitzmann, N.U. Population-Based Linkage of Big Data in Dental Research. *Int. J. Environ. Res. Public Health* **2018**, *15*, 2357–2361. [CrossRef] [PubMed]
11. Boumandjel, N.; Herrmann, F.; Girod, V.; Sieber, C.; Rapin, C.H. Refrigerator content and hospital admission in old people. *Lancet* **2000**, *356*, 563. [CrossRef]
12. Kiss, C.M.; Besimo, C.; Ulrich, A.; Kressig, R.W. Ernährung und Gesundheit im Alter. *Aktuel Ernahrungsmed* **2016**, *41*, 27–35.
13. Majumder, S.; Deen, M.J. Smartphone Sensors for Health Monitoring and Diagnosis. *Sensors* **2019**, *19*, 2164. [CrossRef] [PubMed]
14. Reeder, D.; David, A. Health at hand: A systematic review of smart watch uses for health and wellness. *J. Biomed. Inform.* **2016**, *63*, 269–276. [CrossRef] [PubMed]
15. Beauchet, O.; Blumen, H.M.; Callisaya, M.L.; De Cock, A.M.; Kressig, R.W.; Srikanth, V.; Steinmetz, J.P.; Verghese, J.; Allali, G. Spatiotemporal gait characteristics associated with cognitive impairment: A multicenter cross-sectional study, the intercontinental "Gait, cOgnitiOn & Decline" initiative. *Curr. Alzheimer Res.* **2018**, *23*, 273–282.
16. Brand, C.; Bridenbaugh, A.A.; Perkovac, M.; Glenz, F.; Besimo, C.; Marinello, C.P. The effect of tooth loss on gait stability of community-dwelling older adults. *Gerodontology* **2015**, *32*, 296–301. [CrossRef] [PubMed]
17. Lehne, M.; Sass, J.; Essenwanger, A.; Schepers, J.; Thun, S. Why digital medicine depends on interoperability. *NPJ Digit. Med.* **2019**, *20*, 79. [CrossRef] [PubMed]
18. The Cost of Sequencing a Human Genome. Available online: https://www.genome.gov/about-genomics/fact-sheets/Sequencing-Human-Genome-cost (accessed on 30 October 2019).
19. Payne, K.; Gavan, S.P.; Wright, S.J.; Thompson, A.J. Cost-effectiveness analyses of genetic and genomic diagnostic tests. *Nat. Rev. Genet.* **2018**, *19*, 235–246. [CrossRef] [PubMed]
20. Verordnung (EU) 2016/679 des europäischen Parlaments und des Rates. vom 27. April 2016. zum Schutz natürlicher Personen bei der Verarbeitung personenbezogener Daten, zum freien Datenverkehr und zur Aufhebung der Richtlinie 45/96/EG (Datenschutz-Grundverordnung). Available online: https://eur-lex.europa.eu/eli/reg/2016/679/oj (accessed on 27 April 2016).
21. Hafen, E. Why Citizens Should Have Control of Their Own Data. Available online: https://ethz.ch/en/news-and-events/eth-news/news/2018/04/ernst-hafen-midata.html (accessed on 24 April 2018).
22. Joda, T.; Waltimo, T.; Probst-Hensch, N.; Pauli-Magnus, C.; Zitzmann, N.U. Health data in dentistry: An attempt to master the digital challenge. *Public Health Genom.* **2019**, *22*, 1–7. [CrossRef] [PubMed]
23. Joda, T.; Bornstein, M.M.; Jung, R.E.; Ferrari, M.; Waltimo, T.; Zitzmann, N.U. Recent trends and future direction of dental research in the digital era. *Int. J. Environ. Res. Public Health* **2020**, *17*, 1987. [CrossRef] [PubMed]

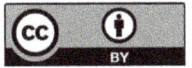

© 2020 by the authors. Licensee MDPI, Basel, Switzerland. This article is an open access article distributed under the terms and conditions of the Creative Commons Attribution (CC BY) license (http://creativecommons.org/licenses/by/4.0/).

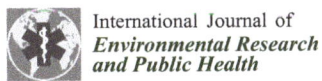

Review

Digital Undergraduate Education in Dentistry: A Systematic Review

Nicola U. Zitzmann *, Lea Matthisson, Harald Ohla and Tim Joda

Department of Reconstructive Dentistry, University Center for Dental Medicine Basel, University of Basel, 4058 Basel, Switzerland; lea.matthisson@unibas.ch (L.M.); h.ohla@unibas.ch (H.O.); tim.joda@unibas.ch (T.J.)
* Correspondence: n.zitzmann@unibas.ch; Tel.: +41-61-267-2636

Received: 23 March 2020; Accepted: 2 May 2020; Published: 7 May 2020

Abstract: The aim of this systematic review was to investigate current penetration and educational quality enhancements from digitalization in the dental curriculum. Using a modified PICO strategy, the literature was searched using PubMed supplemented with a manual search to identify English-language articles published between 1994 and 2020 that reported the use of digital techniques in dental education. A total of 211 articles were identified by electronic search, of which 55 articles were selected for inclusion and supplemented with 27 additional publications retrieved by manual search, resulting in 82 studies that were included in the review. Publications were categorized into five areas of digital dental education: Web-based knowledge transfer and e-learning, digital surface mapping, dental simulator motor skills (including intraoral optical scanning), digital radiography, and surveys related to the penetration and acceptance of digital education. This review demonstrates that digitalization offers great potential to revolutionize dental education to help prepare future dentists for their daily practice. More interactive and intuitive e-learning possibilities will arise to stimulate an enjoyable and meaningful educational experience with 24/7 facilities. Augmented and virtual reality technology will likely play a dominant role in the future of dental education.

Keywords: dental education; digital dentistry; augmented reality (AR); virtual reality (VR)

1. Introduction

The implementation of digital technologies in dental curricula has started globally and reached varying levels of penetration depending on local resources and demands. One of the biggest challenges in digital education is the need to continuously adapt and adjust to the developments in technology and apply these to dental practice [1]. Most dental offices in Europe are equipped with software solutions for managing patients' records, agenda and recall reminders; recording provided services, including working time schedules; ordering materials; and managing the maintenance contracts of medical devices. These systems incorporate medical histories, digital radiographs, intraoral photographs, medicine lists, and correspondences. The systems also enable easy access to detailed odontograms showing fillings per tooth surface, restorations and carious lesions, periodontal status with visualization of the attachment level, probing pocket depth, and recession [2].

The introduction of intraoral optical scanning (IOS) allows the current anatomic situation to be digitized, enabling chairside or laboratory fabrication of restorations, to plan oral rehabilitations with a set-up [3], and/or to superimpose the situation with 3-dimensional (3D) radiography (e.g., for guided implant placement) [4]. While the penetration of these scanners in dental offices is still limited (present in an estimated 20%–25% of European dental offices) [5], laboratory scanners are presumably used by more than two-thirds of dental laboratories. The dental technician uses the 3D model files derived from IOS by the clinician or from scanned conventional casts to facilitate the fabrication of restorations. Compared to waxing, the digital design offers several advantages for quality control, such as providing data about material thickness and values of connector cross sections. While the main shortcomings of lost wax casting were erroneous castings or shrinkage cavities, with a digital workflow the laboratory benefits from improved material properties when industrially manufactured products can be used with subtractive milling or additive printing processes [6].

3D education programs have been introduced to enhance students' spatial ability, their interactivity, critical thinking, and clinical correlations with the integration of multiple dental disciplines. Augmented reality in 3D visualization allows insights in tooth morphology, and also facilitates treatment planning with fixed or removable partial denture (RPD) programs [7]. Digital technologies also include the 3D printing of virtual teeth, which has been suggested to enhance transparency for all students due to the identical setups [8].

A recent review on the application of augmented reality (AR) and virtual reality (VR) in dental medicine demonstrated that the use of AR/VR technologies for educational motor skill training and clinical testing of maxillofacial surgical protocols is increasing [9]. It was concluded that these digital technologies are valuable in dental undergraduate and postgraduate education, offering interactive learning concepts with 24/7 access and objective evaluation. A recent scoping review analyzed the application of VR in pre-clinical dental education and identified four educational thematic areas (simulation hardware, realism of simulation, scoring systems, and validation), highlighting the need for a better evidence base for the utility of VR in dental education [10]. In communicating with dental professionals, medical doctors, dental technicians, and insurance providers, dental students have to be prepared to manage digitized data, ensure patient safety, and understand the benefits and limitations of conventional and digital processes.

Overall, digitalization seems to have had a major impact on dental education, addressing various aspects, such as e-learning and Web-based knowledge transfer, but also related to diagnostics using 3D imaging and digital radiography, and practically oriented trainings in terms of dental simulator motor skills including IOS with 3D printing, prototyping, and digital surface mapping. Digital applications can provide additional opportunities to evaluate and improve education, implementing evidence-based surveys related to the penetration and acceptance of digital education.

The aim of this systematic review was: (i) to investigate the current level of implementation of digital technology in dental education; and (ii) to outline the educational quality enhancements that result from digitalization in main focus areas within the dental curriculum.

2. Materials and Methods

This systematic review was conducted in accordance with the guidelines of Preferred Reporting Items of Systematic Reviews and Meta-Analyses (PRISMA) [11]. A systematic electronic search of PubMed was performed, limited to English-language articles published between 1 January 1994 and 15 April 2020. A modified PICO search was defined for Population/TOPIC, Intervention/METHOD, and Outcome/INTEREST; whereas Comparison was omitted. The search syntax used was: ((students[MeSH]) AND (education, dental[MeSH] OR teaching[MeSH] AND digital)) AND (dentistry[MeSH] OR dental medicine). In addition, the bibliographies of all full texts selected from the electronic search were manually searched, and an extensive search of articles published in the *Journal of Dental Education* and the *European Journal of Dental Education* was conducted.

This systematic review focused on randomized controlled trials, cohort studies, case–control studies, observational trials, and descriptive studies that investigated the application of digital technologies in dental education. Reports without an underlying study design and studies not involving dental students were not included. Furthermore, the vast body of literature about the transition from glass to digital slide microscopy was also excluded. Four reviewers (N.U.Z., T.J., L.M., H.O.) independently screened the titles, abstracts, and the full texts of the identified articles to select those for inclusion in the review. Disagreements were resolved by discussion. Duplicates or preliminary reports that were followed by original publications were excluded.

3. Results

A total of 211 titles were identified by the electronic search (Figure 1). After screening of the titles, abstracts, and full-text articles, 55 publications were included that reported a digital application in dental education. The manual search retrieved 27 additional publications, resulting in the inclusion of 82 studies (Annex S1 and Annex S2).

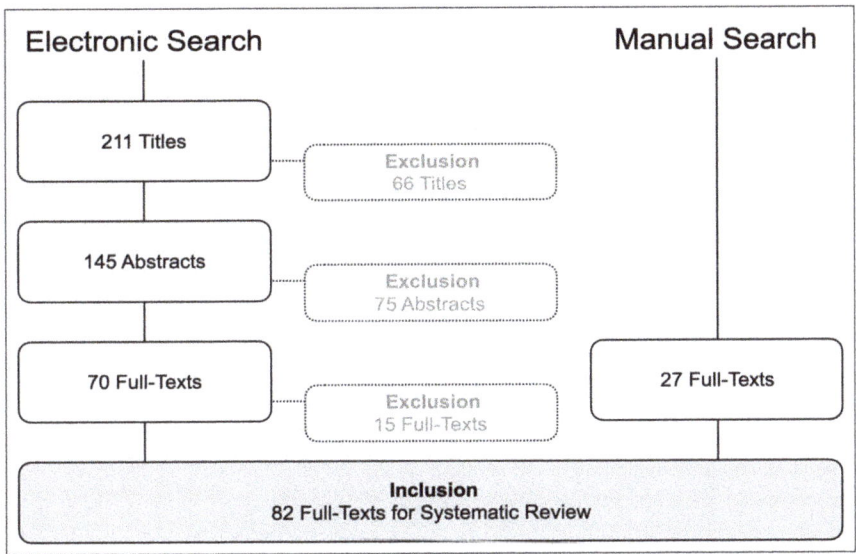

Figure 1. Systematic search strategy.

The publications were categorized into six areas of digital dental education:

- Web-based knowledge transfer/e-learning (22 studies);
- Digital surface mapping (20 studies);
- Dental simulator motor skills including IOS (23 studies);
- 3D printing and prototyping (2 studies);
- Digital radiography (5 studies); and
- Surveys related to the penetration and acceptance of digital education (10 studies).

3.1. Web-Based Knowledge Transfer/e-Learning

Fifteen studies reported the use of Web-based learning tools in the dental curriculum, comprising orthodontics [12,13], tooth anatomy [14–16], oral pathogens and immunology [17], dental radiology [18,19], oral surgery [20] or implant dentistry [21], prosthetic dentistry [22], caries detection [23,24], in growth and development [25], and the general use of Web-based learning tools [26] (Table 1). Three additional studies reported on the use of video illustrations of clinical procedures with behavior management in pediatric dentistry [27], intraoral suturing [28], or tooth preparation [29]. Practicing history-taking and decision-making in periodontology with a Web-based database application, where students used free text communication on the screen to interact with patient data, improved their capability and empathy during the first patient contact [30]. One other study described the introduction of portable digital assistants for undergraduate students in a primary dental care clinic to access a virtual learning environment; these tools proved to be a convenient and versatile method for accessing online education [31]. Mobile devices were found to support learning by offering the opportunity to personalize digital learning materials by making comments, underlining, annotating images, and making drawings [32]. The availability of free 3D viewer software favored the planning of RPD designs on 3D virtual model situations [33]. Online access to digital tools without time restrictions was identified as a major benefit in dental education, and Web-based instructional modules facilitated students' individual learning approach and accommodated varying learning paces. While an initial effort was required to prepare online educational material, faculty time was reduced in the long term.

Table 1. Web-based knowledge transfer / e-learning ($n = 22$).

Study (Year)	Study Design	Theory/Practice	Participants	Materials and Methods	Results
Komolpis et al. 2002 [12]	RCT	P	99	Compared effectiveness (exam scores and time spent) in clinical orthodontic diagnosis in test group (50 students with web-based digital records) and control group (49 students provided with traditional records) with study models, panoramic and cephalometric radiograph, facial and intraoral photographs.	Test and control group performed similar in the exam with no difference in test time; positive feedback about the web-based learning module, students benefit from convenient access to study material on the computer without time constrictions.
Schultze-Mosgau et al. 2004 [20]	OT	T	82	Evaluated a web-based course with a concluding online examination. Feed-back by questionnaire.	Course gradings excellent or good were given for accessibility independent of time (89%), for access independent of location (83%), for objectification of knowledge transfer (67%), and for use of videos for surgical techniques (91%).
Schittek Janda et al. 2004 [30]	RCT	P	39	Compared the effect of a web-based virtual learning environment (VLE) on students' performance in history interview. Both groups underwent standard instruction in professional behavior, history taking, clinical decision making and treatment planning. Test group worked with the virtual periodontal patient for 1 week prior to their first patient contact; control group was first allowed to use the virtual patient after their first patient contact. Time spent, type and order of questions and professional behavior were analyzed.	Test group asked more relevant questions, spent more time on patient issues, and performed a more complete history interview than control. The use of the virtual patient and the process of writing questions in working with the virtual patient stimulated students to organize their knowledge and resulted in more confident behavior towards the patient.
Boynton et al. 2006 [27]	CS	P	108	Explored students' behaviors management in pediatric dentistry using portable video instructions; test group: 11 students reviewing video lecture material on a portable device (iPod) supplementing conventional pediatric behavior management lecture; additional 6 students (intermediate) used audio versions or video on the computer; control group: 91 students without digital learning material; exam on student comprehension.	Test group performed significantly better on the examination (mean 9.3) than control (7.9) or intermediate group (7.8); portable format was preferred.
Reynolds et al. 2007 [31]	CS	P	12	Investigated students' educational use of portable digital assistants (PDA) to access a Virtual Learning Environment in a primary dentalcare clinic and at home; cross over trial with 6 students with / 6 without for 12 weeks.	PDA was frequently used for online education; over 90% wanted PDA as part of their dental kit.
Kingsley et al. 2009 [17]	CS	P	78	Examined students' ability to use web-based online technologies to find recently published online citations and to answer clinically relevant questions (oral pathogens and immunology course); technology skills analyzed: ability to locate online library resources, understand how information is organized within the library system, access online databases, interpret and evaluate research materials within the context of a specific discipline; students were provided with a review article of vaccines against caries from 2001.	100% of students had correct responses to the content-specific or technology-independent portions; 46% had correct responses to the information literacy or technology-dependent portions; as web-based technologies grow more prevalent in the digital era, information literacy and technology-dependent, applied research assignments should be integrated into graduate-level curricula.
Weaver et al. 2009 [28]	RCT	P	12	Evaluated performance in intraoral suturing after digital multimedia instruction; control group: written information; test group: plus teaching tool; suturing performed on a model situation, evaluated by 10 grading criteria.	Test group performed better than control; video addressed common mistakes made by novice students, improved long-term understanding of the basic suture principles.

Table 1. Cont.

Study (Year)	Study Design	Theory/Practice	Participants	Materials and Methods	Results
Wright et al. 2009 [14]	OT	T	235	Determined whether dental students used an interactive DVD-tooth atlas as a study aid and perceived the 3D interactive tooth atlas as a value-added learning experience.	14% students downloaded the DVD voluntarily prior to adding atlas-related exam questions as incentives; after adding incentives 43% downloaded the material; financial concerns and overly sophisticated content were deemed responsible for the low acceptance.
Curnier 2010 [16]	OT	P	26	Assessed VR integration into teaching of dental anatomy, feedback by questionnaire	70% of the students were satisfied/very satisfied with IT integration in the curriculum.
Bains et al. 2010 [13]	RCT	T	90	Compared effectiveness and attitudes toward e-learning (EL, online tutorial without teacher), face-to-face learning (F2FL, led by teacher) and blended learning (BL) subdivided in BL1 (EL first then F2FL) and BL2 (F2FL first then EL) among 4th year students. Groups received cephalometric tutorial in the allocated mode, answered an MCQ (Multiple Choice Questionnaire).	F2FL and BL resulted in similar test results; EL alone was less effective. BL was the most and F2FL was the least accepted method, EL was significantly less preferred, the order B1 or 2 had no effect.
Mitov et al. 2010 [15]	CS	T	36	Testing an e-learning software (morphoDent) to prepare for an anatomy exam. 3D models with description and x-rays of permanent human teeth were available for viewing and interaction on the learning platform. Practical dental morphology exam was compared to virtual tooth anatomy exam. Evaluation of students' perceptions in a questionnaire.	Similar exam scores in traditional and online exam. Majority felt the software helped them learning dental morphology, despite of difficulties in operating the program.
Vuchkova et al. 2012 [19]	CS	P	88	Evaluated interactive digital versus conventional radiology textbook (course radiographic anatomy), outcome was radiographic interpretation test and survey feedback.	95% perceived positive enhancement of learning and interpretation.
Smith et al. 2012 [29]	OT	P	26	Compared the use of online video-clips with traditional live demonstrations with one-to-one supervision; students exam scores before and after the video introduction were compared. Feed-back by questionnaire.	76% preferred video-clips to live demonstrations, 57% reviewed DVD at home; 57% felt one-to-one supervision more effective developing their competence in tooth preparation.
Qi et al. 2013 [21]	RCT	P	95	Comparison of active versus passive approaches in using 3D virtual scenes in dental implant cases. Students were exposed to educational materials about implant restoration on three types of webpages: traditional 2D (group 1); active-controlling 3D (group 2); passive-controlling 3D (group 3). After reviewing their webpages, students were asked to complete a posttest to assess the relative quality of information acquisition. Before study exposure, students performed a standardized test of spatial ability (mental rotations test, MRT).	Posttest scores were highest in group 3 (passive control) and lowest in group 2 (active control). Higher MRT scores were associated with better posttest performances in all three groups. Individuals with low spatial ability did not benefit from 3D interactive virtual reality, while passive control produced higher learning effects compared to active control.
Reissmann et al. 2015 [22]	OT	T	71	Creation of a blended learning model; e-learning modules covered fundamental principles, additional information, and learning tests (tests were repeated until passed and the next video sequence unlocked); modules comprised (i) tooth preparation, placement of post and core, and provisional crown; (ii) with preparation, manufacturing and insertion of a FDP (Fixed Dental Prosthesis). Students rated the course on a questionnaire, comparison to previous courses without e-learning.	Significantly higher satisfaction among students enrolled in the e-learning modules compared to the years prior to integration of the e-learning tests. Results suggest that instructor-based practical demonstrations in preclinical courses in prosthetic dentistry could be successfully replaced by e-learning applications provided that course content is structured according to specific predefined learning goals and procedures.
Luz et al. 2015 [24]	RCT	P	39	Evaluated the effect of a digital learning tool on students' caries detection in 12 pediatric patients (3.4 per student) using ICDAS (International Caries Detection & Assessment System) (1264 dental surfaces). 2 weeks after first exam students were split into 3 training groups: Group 1: ICDAS e-learning program; group 2: plus digital learning tool; group 3: no learning strategy; students reassessed the same patients 2 weeks, and results compared.	After training group 1 and 2 had improved with significantly higher sensitivity; group 2 showed significant increase in sensitivity at the D2 and D3 thresholds as a result of the digital learning tool.

Table 1. *Cont.*

Study (Year)	Study Design	Theory/Practice	Participants	Materials and Methods	Results
Gonzales et al. 2016 [18]	OT	T	40	Implementation social media (Twitter) in a dental radiology course and evaluated students' use and perception by a questionnaire.	95% (38) had not used Twitter prior to the course; 53% (21) created an account during the course to view radiographic examples and stay informed; overall Twitter had a positive impact with improved accessibility to the instructor.
Jackson et al. 2018 [25]	OT	P	80	Evaluated dental students study patterns using self-directed web-based learning modules with scheduled self-study time instead of lectures; web-based module access (date and time) was recorded for four courses in the growth & development curriculum; scheduled access time was 8 am to 5 pm.	Frequency of module access (at least once) varied among the four courses (10–64%); only three students had > 20% of their total accesses taking place during designated self-study times. For all courses the proportion of module access was significantly higher 0–2 days before an exam compared to 3–7 or >7 days before final exam; no association between module access during scheduled times and course performance.
Alves et al. 2018 [23]	RCT	P	64	Evaluated the effect of a digital learning tool on students' caries detection in 80 teeth using ICDAS; Group 1 (21 students): ICDAS e-learning program; group 2 (22 students): plus digital learning tool; group 3 (21 students): no training; reassessment of the 80 teeth 2 weeks after training.	After training group 1 and 2 had improved with significantly higher sensitivity and specificity; group 3 had increased sensitivity at the D2 thresholds; ICDAS e-learning with or without digital learning tool improved occlusal caries detection.
Botelho et al. 2019 [26]	OT	T	40	Surveyed dental students' perception of cloud-based practice records (documenting clinical progression) compared to traditional paper record.	Cloud based records were rated significantly better in terms of usefulness, ease of use, and learning, satisfaction.
Pyörälä et al. 2019 [32]	OT	T	176	Investigated perception of mobile devices for study use among 124 medical, 52 dental students provided with iPads and followed from 1st to 5th year; feed-back by questionnaire.	Note taking was the most frequent application of the mobile device in the 1st–5th year; students personalized digital learning materials by making comments, underlining, marking images and drawings. Students retrieved their notes anytime when studying for examinations and treating patients in clinical practice.
Mahrous et al. 2019 [33]	RCT	P	77	Compared virtual 3D casts with 2D paper-based exercise in planning removable partial denture design; group 1 ($n = 39$) planned RPD in Kennedy class IV in virtual 3D and Kennedy class II in traditional 2D format, group 2 (=38) planned class IV traditional and class II virtual; survey lines and undercut positions were drawn on virtual 3D casts or given in written descriptions (2D); students planned design (with rests, clasp type, retention location, guide plane) was scored; feed-back by questionnaire.	Similar scores for 3D and 2D exercises; majority favored virtual 3D casts because of improved understanding of relevant parameters and spatial visualization. Currently, physical casts are still required to practice surveying and drawing on the cast.

RCT = Randomized Controlled Trial; CT = Controlled Trial; CS = Cohort Study; CCS = Case-Control-Study; OT = Observational Study.

3.2. Digital Surface Mapping

Visual inspection of students' work is known to have shortcomings in inter- and intra-examiner reliability, whereas standardized digital surface mapping of abutment tooth preparations facilitates objective evaluation and feedback (Table 2) [34–46]. In the preclinical training of dental students, the use of software that can match the student's scanned preparation with an ideal tooth preparation has been proven to be a helpful tool in the evaluation of preparation form, taper, and substance removal. High intra-rater agreement was also found for the repeated digital grading of wax-ups in the undergraduate curriculum [47], and students' initial self-assessment was overrated compared to the digital grading [48]. Limitations of digital assessments have been found for intracoronal cavity preparations, due to the restricted analysis of cavity depth [49,50]. With specified software skills, successful application was documented for class II mesio-occlusal-distal (MOD) cavity assessments, class III composite preparations, and mesio-occlusal (MO) onlay preparations [51–53]. These studies of digital surface mapping clearly demonstrate the tremendous development of this technology since 2006, which now enables a thorough and consistent analysis of several preparation parameters, with freely available open-source comparison tools.

Table 2. Digital surface mapping (n = 20).

Study (Year)	Study Design	Theory/Practice	Participants	Materials and Methods	Results
Esser et al. 2006 [35]	CS	P	36	Compared conventional visual examination by faculty with digital analysis ("Prep Assistant") of students' preparation of a central incisor for a metal-ceramic crown; preparations were scanned; before the exam preparation, students had received theoretical and practical exercises.	Digital measuring technique was superior for convergence angle, occlusal reduction and width of shoulder; low correlation between visual and digital was observed for the assessments of chamfer, path of insertion, width of bevel and basic form; calibration of evaluators benefit from digital analysis tool.
Hamil et al. 2014 [37]	OT	P	81	Evaluated dental students' opinion about a new grading software program (E4D Compare with surface mapping technology) for their self-assessment and as faculty-grading tool in a preclinical course to evaluate crown preparations. Software was introduced (one-hour lecture and three-hour hands-on laboratory session) and applied for self-assessment during one semester; questionnaire about students' perception.	Students preferred digital grading system over traditional hand-grading 95% reported on feedback inconsistencies among different faculty members, 72% reported on inconsistencies from the examiner; 85% agreed or strongly agreed that E4D Compare provided more consistent grading than faculty; 79% responded that the software provided more feedback, 90% found the software helping them to understand their deficiencies; 89% agreed or strongly agreed that E4D Compare grading helped them be better clinicians.
Mays et al. 2014 [49]	CT	P	25	Compared students' visual self-assessment, students' digital (CAD/CAM) self-assessment, faculty visual assessment, and faculty digital assessment. Students prepared mesial-occlusal amalgam cavity, used standardized grading sheets for visual self-assessment, scanned their preparation, used design tool of Cerec software for digital self-assessment.	Moderate agreement between faculty visual and digital evaluation for occlusal and proximal shape, orientation and definition; poor agreement between student visual and digital evaluation for occlusal shape, and fair for proximal shape, orientation and definition; slight to poor agreement between students visual and faculty visual evaluation, and digital assessment did not improve student/faculty agreement.
Kwon et al. 2014 [47]	OT	P	60	Compared conventional visual faculty grading of wax-ups to digital assessment in dental anatomy course; 30 faculty wax-ups, 15 student wax-ups and 15 dentoform teeth; visual grading was performed by two experienced faculty members, digital grading by one operator, both gradings were repeated after 1 week; maxillary 1st molar wax-up (from faculty) with highest scores from visual grading was used as master model for digital grading.	Modest intra-rater reliability for visual scoring with similar rating between the two trials (0.7); low inter-rater agreement between the two faculty raters; digital grading showed high intra-rater agreement for the repeated assessment (ICC 0.9); modest correlation between visual and digital grading.
Garrett et al. 2015 [48]	CCS	P	57	Evaluated E4D software (Planmeca) to assess incisor and molar wax-ups of 57 students, who used digital images for self-assessment, and compare to faculty members; based on five assessment criteria (arch alignment, proximal contacts, proximal contour and embrasures, facial contour, lingual contour) and applying 300, 400, and 500 µm level of tolerance in E4D.	Students' self-assessment of the maxillary incisor wax-up was higher than faculty and E4D300, but lower than E4D 400 and 500. For the molar wax-up, self-assessment was not different to faculty, but higher than E4D300. E4D500 evaluations were sig. superior than other assessments.

Table 2. *Cont.*

Study (Year)	Study Design	Theory/Practice	Participants	Materials and Methods	Results
Callan et al. 2015 [34]	CCS	P	82	Validated E4D software (Planmeca) to assess molar crown preparation of 82 students and compare to calibrated faculty members based on four criteria (occlusal reduction, proximal reduction, facial/lingual reduction, margins and draw). Agreement in rankings between faculty scores and E4D Compare scores was measured with Spearman's correlation coefficient (SCC) at five different tolerance levels (0.1–0.5 mm).	SCC values for practical exams varied between 0.20 and 0.56. None of the upper 95% confidence limits reached the for strong correlation. SCC values indicated only weak to moderate agreement in ranks between practical exam scores and scores obtained with E4D Compare. When ranked from lowest to highest, the results from the conventional grading by the faculty did not correlate within an acceptable range to E4D Compare software data.
Mays et al. 2016 [42]	CCS	P	50	Validated E4D software (Planmeca) to assess occlusal convergence (TOC) of 50 molar crown preparations from students and compared to traditional faculty assessment.	Digital software could distinguish differences in TOC, which were grouped as minimum taper (mean 11°), moderate (mean 23°), or excessive (mean 47°). Digital TOC evaluation was more objective compared to faculty visual scoring.
Gratton et al. 2016 [45]	RCT	P	80	Compared effect of access to digital systems in addition to conventional preparation instructions; CEREC prepCheck ($n = 20$), E4D Compare ($n=20$), and control without access to digital system ($n = 40$); incisor and molar crown preparations were assessed by the students, by 3 faculties and by E4D Compare at 0.30 mm tolerance.	All groups had similar preparation scores. Visual and digital assessment scores showed modest correlation.
Gratton et al. 2017 [46]	RCT	P	79	Compared digital systems Compare ($n = 42$) and prepCheck ($n = 37$) as additional evaluation tool assessing their crown preparations (maxillary central incisor and mandibular molar); all preparations were graded by faculty Compare and prepCheck; feed-back with post-course questionnaire.	Both groups had similar technical scores; both systems had modest correlation with faculty scores and strong correlation with each other. 55.3% of students felt unfavorable about learning digital evaluation protocols, while 62.3% felt favorable about the integration of the tools into the curriculum.
Park et al. 2017 [44]	OT	P	36	Evaluated prepCheck for self-assessment, students performed ceramo-metal crown preparation (maxillary molar during formative exercise, mandibular molar during summative exam); five learning tools were used for assessments: reduction, margin width, surface finish, taper, undercut; tools were rated for usefulness, user-friendliness, and frequency of use (scale from 1 = lowest to 5 = highest). Faculty members graded tooth preparations as pass (P), marginal-pass (MP), or fail (F).	Tools assessing undercut and taper received highest scores for usefulness, user-friendliness, and frequency of use. Students' performance was 38.8% P, 30.6% MP and 30.6% F. Failing students had the highest score (4.4) on usefulness.
Kateeb et al. 2017 [38]	OT	P	96	Compared digital assessment software of students' crown preparation with traditional visual inspection; four examiners; sample of 20 preparations were reassessed for intra-rater reliability.	Intra-rater reliability (ICC) was 0.73–0.78 and 0.99 for the digital grading system; inter-rater reliability among the four examiners was good (0.76); agreement between examiners and digital ratings were low to moderate; digital grading was more consistent.
Sly et al. 2017 [50]	OT	P	98	Compared E4D software (Planmeca) to assess students intracoronal Class I preparation with traditional visual inspection; four examiners.	Similar results for grading of isthmus width and remaining marginal ridge, while pulpal floor depth was assessed more precisely with visual inspection; results indicate that software has limitations for intracoronal cavity assessment but offers a self-assessment tool to improve psychomotor skills with independent and immediate feedback.
Kunkel et al. 2018 [40]	OT	P	69	Compared prepCheck with visual faculty assessment of taper in students' crown preparation of typodont teeth, 10 experienced course instructors.	Instructor gradings were overrated compared to digital prepCheck grades, prepCheck facilitates evaluation instantly and exactly by students and examiners.

Table 2. Cont.

Study (Year)	Study Design	Theory/Practice	Participants	Materials and Methods	Results
Kozarovska & Larsson 2018 [39]	RCT	P	57	Evaluated a digital preparation validation tool (PVT) for students' self-assessment of crown preparation (tooth 11 and 21); group A ("prep-and-scan" self-assessed and scanned three preparations; group B ("best-of-three") self-assessed the three attempts, chose the best for scanning; questionnaire about students' and teachers' experiences with PVT.	Group A showed an increase in agreement of self-assessment and feedback from PVT, while group B showed low level agreement with PVT. Bucco-incisal reduction, reduction of the tuberculum surface and presence of undercuts were difficult to correctly identify by the students. Questionnaire feedback revealed need for PVT to develop skills, to ease assessment, while critical aspects were PVT's time efficiency and the need for verbal feedback. Teachers observed the PVT as a motivation during skills laboratory training, while verbal feedback were still deemed necessary.
Wolgin et al. 2018 [53]	RCT	P	47	Investigated digital self-assessment concept (prepCheck software) for students in the phantom course preparing a three surface (MOD) class II amalgam cavity; intervention group (IG): compared a 3D image of their preparation against master preparation with PrepCheck; control group (CG): received verbal feedback from supervisor based on pre-defined criteria.	Test and control groups performed similar and self-assessment learning tool was deemed equivalent to conventional supervision.
Lee et al. 2018 [51]	OT	P	69	Compared students' self-assessment (conventional and digital with Cerec software) with assessment (conventional and digital) by faculty members for class II amalgam preparations (C2AP) and Class III composite preparations (C3CP).	Students overestimated their performance (positive S-F gap) in both the C2AP and C3CP preparation exercises in conventional (11% and 5%) and digital assessments (8% and 2%); in conventional assessments, preclinical performance was negatively correlated with student-faculty gap ($r = -0.47$, $p < 0.001$); particularly students in the bottom quartile sig. improved their self-assessment accuracy using digital self-assessments over conventional assessments.
Nagy et al. 2018 [52]	RCT	P	36	Investigated the effect of a digital feedback (test group) for mesio-occlusal onlay preparation by a 3D visualization of the cavity (Dental Teacher software, KaVo), while verbal feedback from supervisor was given to control group. Following feedbacks, 2nd corrective preparations were conducted and improvements measured. Parameters: occlusal cavity depth (OD), approximal depth (AD), extent of cusp reduction on the mesiobuccal cusp (CR), width of shoulder preparation around the mesiobuccal cusp (SW), cavity width at two different points in the occlusal box (OW).	Test group improved in all parameter and showed significantly smaller deviations of mean OD, AD and mean SW; in control group, parameter deviations were similar during 1st and 2nd preparation.
Liu et al. 2018 [41]	RCT	P	66	Evaluated the effectiveness of preclinical training on ceramic crown preparation using digital training system compared with traditional training method; test group: trained with digital method with Online Peer-Review System (OPRS) and Real-time Dental Training and Evaluation System (RDTES); control group: traditional method with instructor demonstration and evaluation; central incisor crown preparation.	Five of 15 assessed items were significantly better in test group; 96.97% of test students agreed or strongly agreed that using digital training system could better improve the practical ability than traditional method.
Greany et al. 2019 [36]	OT	P	67	Compared conventional visual faculty inspection of wax-ups to digital assessment; six examiners evaluated 67 students' wax-ups of maxillary first molar, reevaluation after 1 week; scan with IOS, STL files imported to free available open source data cloud comparison utility (Cloud Compare.org), digital evaluation by two examiners.	Visual inspection had low inter-examiner precision (ICC 0.332) and accuracy; intra-examiner precision for reevaluation was low; inter-examiner precision of digital exam was high (ICC 0.866) with high accuracy.

Table 2. *Cont.*

Study (Year)	Study Design	Theory/Practice	Participants	Materials and Methods	Results
Miyazone et al. 2019 [43]	OT	P	100	Compared prepCheck with visual faculty assessment of students' crown preparation of typodont teeth (mandibular first molar as crown abutment, maxillary 2nd premolar and 2nd molar as FDP abutments), assess inter- and intra-grader agreement of five experienced examiners conducting visual and digital exam; scoring repeated three times; parameters for crown abutments: axial tissue removal, margin width, undercut, occlusal reduction, cusp tips, occlusal anatomy; for FDP abutments: path of insertion.	Intra-grader agreement was better with prepCheck than visual assessment for all parameters except cusp tip and occlusal anatomy; inter-grader agreement for path of insertion was questionable with visual, but good with digital assessment. Inter-grader disagreement was greater in visual than digital assessment. Overestimation of tooth reduction in visual grading was eliminated by digital analysis.

RCT = Randomized Controlled Trial; CT = Controlled Trial; CS = Cohort Study; CCS = Case-Control-Study; OT = Observational Study; ICC = Inter-Class Correlation; STL = Standard Tessellation Language.

3.3. Dental Simulator Motor Skills Including Intraoral Optical Scanning

A high level of interest and acceptance was documented among undergraduate students for simulator training in cavity preparations [54–56], or in surgical interventions such as apicoectomies (Table 3) [57]. A trend toward improved technical skills and ergonomics was documented when simulator training with real-time feedback was added to traditional instructions [58–60]. Training with a VR-based simulator improved students' preparation of class I occlusal cavities [61], and of abutments for porcelain-fused-to-metal crowns [62]. In evaluating the manual dexterity of students, professionals, and non-professionals, the simulator scoring algorithm showed a high reliability to differentiate between non-professionals and dental students or dentists [63]. Instruction time from faculty for teaching cavity and crown preparations was significantly reduced when virtual reality computer-assisted simulation systems were used compared to contemporary non-computer-assisted simulation systems [64]. Preparation performance on VR units with continuous evaluations and advice from clinical instructors led to better preparation quality than real-time feedback from the virtual dental unit. Self-paced learning and the immediate software feedback were beneficial with the VR unit, and it was perceived as adjunct, but not replacing faculty instructions [65]. Students requested software improvements with more realistic force feedback during interaction with different tissues in the virtual oral environment including the maxilla, mandible, gum, tongue, cheek, enamel, dentine, pulp, cementum, etc. [66]. Recent advancements of simulators enabled variations in force feedback accounting for varying hardness of the virtual material, cut speed gain, and push force [67].

Improved student performance in crown digitization and framework design was observed when CAD/CAM (Computer-Aided Design/ Computer-aided manufacturing) courses were introduced in dental education [68]. While students enjoyed designing a full crown using CAD as compared to traditional waxing, limits of the technology in representing anatomic contours and excursive occlusion were identified [69]. Viewing their scanned crown preparations magnified on the screen improved students' understanding of the finishing line [70]. The application of IOS in the simulation training showed that even inexperienced dental students were capable of acquiring the skills needed to use digital tools, and students preferred IOS over conventional impressions [71,72]. Furthermore, students' work time was shorter with IOS than with conventional impression [72,73], although more teaching time was required for digital scanning than for conventional impression techniques [74]. Applying digital complete denture treatment (AvaDent; AvaDent Digital Dental Solutions, Scottsdale, AZ, USA) in the student clinics resulted in restorations with superior gradings that were preferred by both students and patients [75]. Using an intraoral camera increased patients' consent for crown treatment, and was positively perceived by students and patients, while faculty members were neutral [76].

Table 3. Dental simulator motor skills incl. IOS ($n = 23$).

Study (Year)	Study Design	Theory / Practice	Participants	Materials and Methods	Results
Quinn et al. 2003 [65]	RCT	P	20	Compared students' performance in preparing class I amalgam cavity on a VR-based training unit; test group had virtual real-time feedback and software evaluation, control group had clinical instructor available during preparation. Anonymous scoring by 2 faculties, criteria: outline form, retention form, smoothness, cavity depth and cavity margin angulation. Questionnaire feed-back in test group.	Similar results for retention and wall angulation, while outline form, smoothness and cavity depth scored better in control. Test group assessed software as superior for immediate feed-back, self-paced learning, consistency of evaluation, encouraging independent work and more thorough assessment, while conventional training was superior for increasing confidence in cavity preparation. VR-based training should be used as adjunct but not replacing conventional training methods.
Jasinevicius et al. 2004 [64]	CT	P	28	Compared students' performance in amalgam and crown preparations on typodont teeth either with a contemporary non-computer-assisted simulation system (CS), or with a virtual reality computer-assisted simulation system (VR). Both groups were provided with presentations describing preparations, CS group received handouts, VR group had preparation criteria available on the computer. Student-faculty (S-F) interaction time was logged.	Preparation quality did not differ between CS and VR. CS required 2.8 h, VR 0.5 h S-F. CS received five times more instructional time from faculty than VR.
LeBlanc et al. 2004 [60]	RCT	P	68	Compared students' technical skills in preclinical operative dentistry after standard traditional laboratory-based instructions (over 110 h) and additional virtual reality simulator-enhanced training (test group with 20 students) Simulator (DentSim, DenX) provided real-time feedback, training conducted during 6–10 h in 3 blocks over 8 months.	While all students improved in the 4 tests during the year, test students tended to better scores in the final exam. Virtual reality simulators can be implemented in the traditional training of future dentists.
Rees et al. 2007 [54]	CT	P	16	Evaluated simulator training (DentSim, DenX) by undergraduate students for Class I and II preparations (time, marks, number of evaluations), students spent 6 h cutting an unlimited number of Class I cavities and Class II cavities; feedback by questionnaire.	Class I preparations obtained a mean mark of 66.8, preparation time was 12.5 min, with 6.7 evaluations; Class II had a mark of 26.5, time 18 min, with 7.0 evaluations. Class II was more difficult to cut. Students appreciated easy change of teeth, working at their own pace and examine the cavity in a cross-section.
Welk et al. 2008 [55]	OT	P/T	80	Evaluated students' performance in operative dentistry after training with computer-assisted dental simulator (DentSim, DenX), feedback by questionnaire.	Students indicated high interest in simulator training, high acceptance and response to additional elective training time in the computer assisted simulation lab. The shift in curriculum and instructional goals has to be optimized continuously.
Urbankova et al. 2010 [58]	RCT	P	75	Evaluated adjunctive computerized dental simulator (CDS; DentSim) training (8 h) in operative dentistry (Class I and II preparations): either before ($n = 26$) or after 1st exam ($n = 13$); control group ($n = 36$) with traditional preclinical dental training alone (110 h).	CDS-trained students performed better than control in the 1st and 2nd exam, no difference between pre-exam and post-exam groups. In the 3rd exam (end of the year) CDS group had higher, but not significantly different scores than control.
Pohlenz et al. 2010 [57]	CT	P	53	Evaluated VR training (Voxel-Man) for virtual apicoectomy; questionnaire about simulated force feedback, spatial 3D perception, resolution and integration of further pathologic conditions.	92.7% recommended the virtual simulation as additional modality in dental education, 81.1% reported the simulated force feedback as good or very good, 86.8% evaluated 3D spatial perception as good or very good; 100% recommended integration of further pathologies.

Table 3. Cont.

Study (Year)	Study Design	Theory / Practice	Participants	Materials and Methods	Results
Gottlieb et al. 2011 [59]	CT	T	202	Evaluated VR simulation training (DentSim, Image Navigation Ltd.) in operative preparations and restorations, 60 h VR training, laboratory course was reduced to 234 h (instead of traditional 304h). 13 experienced faculties assessed 97 non-VR students (1st year, control) and 105 students with 1 semester VR experience (test); survey about students' abilities in ergonomics, confidence level, performance, preparation, and self-assessment.	Faculty expected greater psychomotor skills and ability to prepare teeth in VR, abilities were lower than anticipated but numerically higher than in non-VR students. Faculty members perceived students' ergonomics in the test group better than in control.
Ben-Gal et al. 2011 [56]	CT	P	33	Evaluated use of VR simulator (IDEA Dental) for dental instruction, self-practice, and student evaluation. 21 experienced dental educators, 12 randomly selected experienced dental students (5th year) performed 5 drilling tasks using the simulator, feed-back by questionnaire.	Both groups found that the simulator could provide significant benefits in teaching and self-learning of manual dental skills.
Ben-Gal et al. 2013 [63]	CT	P	106	Evaluated potential of VR training simulator (IDEA Dental) to assess manual dexterity in 63 dental students, 28 dentists, 14 non-dentists, performed virtual drilling tasks in different geometric shapes: time to completion, accuracy, number of trials to successful completion, score provided by the simulator.	Simulator scoring algorithm showed high reliability in all parameters and was able to differentiate between non-professionals and dental students or non-professionals and dentists.
Lee & Gallucci 2013 [73]	CT	P	30	Compared digital (IOS) to conventional impression for single implant restorations, evaluated efficiency, difficulty and students' preference.	Mean total treatment time, preparation time and working time were significantly longer for conventional than for IOS; conventional impressions were assessed as more difficult than IOS; 60% preferred IOS, 7% conventional, 33% either techniques
Kikuchi et al. 2013 [62]	RCT	P	43	Compared VR simulator (DentSim) training with or without instructor feedback for preparation of porcelain fused to metal (PFM) crown preparation. 43 students (5th year). randomly divided into: 1. VR group with instructor's feedback (DSF; $n = 15$); 2. VR without instructor's feedback (DS; $n = 15$); 3. neither VR simulator training nor faculty feedback (NDS; $n = 13$); preparation time and scores of 4 crown preparations (1 week for 4 weeks).	DSF and DS had significantly higher total scores than NDS. Similar results in DSF and DS, but shortened preparation time with instructors' feed-back (DSF) at early stages.
Douglas et al. 2014 [69]	CT	P	50	Compared students' performance in traditional waxing vs. computer-aided crown designing (IOS with CEREC 3D, Sirona Dental Systems), faculty grading of occlusal contacts and anatomic form, feed-back by questionnaire.	Similar gradings for wax design (79.1) and crown design (78.3); more occlusal contacts with CAD; students enjoyed designing a full contour crown using CAD and required less time with CAD. Students recognized limits of CAD technology in representing anatomic contours and excursive occlusion compared to conventional wax techniques.
Wang et al. 2015 [66]	CT	P	20	Compared VR simulator (iDental with Phanotm Omni, SensAble Tech. Inc.) in novice group (graduate students with less than 3 years clinical practice experience) and resident group (with 3–0 years clinical practice); assessment of caries removal, pulp chamber opening, time and amount of removed healthy/unhealthy tissue; feed-back by a questionnaire.	No differences in time and amount of tissue removal between groups; residents spend slightly more time than students; both groups suggested improvements in spatial registration precision, more realistic model with material properties and force feedback of different tissues, improvement of the depth of the virtual space.
Schwindling et al. 2015 [68]	CT	P	56	Evaluated a CAD/CAM hands-on course (test) compared to video-supported lecture only (control); written exam about cast digitizing and zirconia crown designing.	Test group performed significantly better than controls (16.8/20 vs. 12.5/20 correct answers); interest of students in CAD/CAM was higher after hands-on course.
Kattadiyil et al. 2015 [75]	CCS	P	15	Compared clinical treatment outcomes, patient satisfaction, and dental student preferences for digital (AvaDent, two appointments) and conventional (five appointments) complete dentures (CD) in 15 patients, 15 dental students fabricated two sets of CDs for each patient. Faculty and patient ratings, patient and student preferences, perceptions, treatment time was analyzed.	Digital process was equally effective and more time-efficient than conventional; faculty scored digital better than conventional dentures; patients and students preferred digital dentures.

Table 3. *Cont.*

Study (Year)	Study Design	Theory/Practice	Participants	Materials and Methods	Results
Zitzmann et al. 2017 [72]	RCT	P	50	Investigated performance (time recording) and perception (questionnaire feedback) of IOS and conventional implant impression after video teaching.	Students rated conventional impressions as more difficult (VAS 46) than IOS (VAS 70), with greater patient-friendliness of IOS (VAS 83) compared to conventional impressions (VAS 36); 76% preferred digital, 88% felt most effective with IOS; total work time of all steps was significantly shorter with 301 sec. for IOS and 723 sec. for conventional impressions.
Wegner et al. 2017 [70]	OT	P	108	Evaluated students' perception (questionnaire feedback) of IOS (Lava Cos Training, 3M Espe), scanning of 3 typodont tooth preparations.	63.9% positive opinion, 60.2% considered scanning process as manageable, 55.6% profited from magnified view of their preparation to understand chamfer finish lines.
Marti et al. 2017 [74]	RCT	P	25	Analyzed time to instruct IOS (DS; LAVA C.O.S. digital impression system) and conventional impression technique (CI; polyvinyl siloxane) with video lecture, investigator led demonstration, and independent impression exercise; time recording and questionnaire about familiarity and student's expectations.	Teaching DS required significantly more time than CI for video lecture (16 vs. 10 min), demonstration time (9 vs 5 min) and impression time (18 vs. 9 min). Initially students were more familiar with CI (3.96) than DS (1.96) technique. After instructions and practice, CI technique proved significantly easier than expected. Manageability of DS was not influenced by the instruction and practice experience. 96% expressed an expectation that DS will become their predominant impression technique.
de Boer et al. 2019 [67]	RCT	P	126	Investigated skill transfer between various levels of force feedback (FFB) using Simodont dental trainer (Moog) for cross-figure preparations as manual dexterity exercise. Assessment of students' satisfaction by questionnaire.	Longer practice time was correlated with test performance: students passing at different FFB levels had mean of 300h, those passing in one FFB level had 271 h, failing students had 224 h. Skill transfer from one level of FFB to another was feasible with sufficient training.
Schott et al. 2019 [71]	OT	P	31	Evaluated dental students' perception of IOS compared to conventional alginate impression; survey after basic training and self-practicing.	77% (24) students were overall "very" or "rather satisfied" with the handling of IOS; 58% preferred IOS from the dentist's perspective, no significant difference from the patient's perspective but reduced comfort related to the impression tray.
Murbay et al. 2020 [61]	RCT	P	32	Incorporated VR with Moog Simodont dental trainer in preclinical training; students performed an occlusal preparation on typodont teeth and had previous exposure to VR (group 1) or no VR exposure (group 2); assessment was conducted (satisfactory / unsatisfactory) by manual approach or digital (Magic 19.01 64-bit).	VR use improved preparation significantly with 75% (12/16) satisfactory preparations in group 1 and 44% (7/16) in group 2. Manual and digital evaluation methods did not differ significantly.
Murrell et al. 2019 [76]	OT	P	288	Evaluated completion of posterior crown planning with or without presenting the situation to the patient by intraoral camera use; 51 students completed 198 surveys, 35 faculty members with 64 surveys, 202 patient surveys, survey was voluntary and camera use optional.	Positive perception of intraoral camera use by students and patients, while faculty was neutral; significantly higher completion rate when intraoral camera was used.

RCT = Randomized Controlled Trial; CT = Controlled Trial; CS = Cohort Study; CCS = Case-Control-Study; OT = Observational Study; DSF = VR group with instructor feedback; DS = VR group without instructor feedback; NDS = Neither VR simulator training nor faculty feedback; VAS = Visual Analog Scale; IDEA = International Dental Education Association.

3.4. 3D Rapid Prototyping

Two studies evaluated training models created by 3D rapid prototyping [77,78]. Such methods can supplement teaching on human teeth or even replace it, and educational needs can easily be adapted to students' skills (Table 4).

Table 4. Group 4: 3D printing and prototyping ($n = 2$).

Study (Year)	Study Design	Theory/Practice	Participants	Materials and Methods	Results
Soares et al. 2013 [77]	OT	T	40	Cavity preparation was taught with conventional teaching materials with 2D schematic illustration and photographs. New didactic material with virtual 3D (videos of the preparations) and magnified nylon prototyped models was introduced. Evaluation by questionnaire.	Improvement of teaching quality when combining 3D virtual technology with real models.
Kröger et al. 2016 [78]	OT	P	22	3D printed simulation models based on real patient situations were used for hands-on practice. Models simulated realistic tooth positions and wide variability of dental cases and procedures. Students removed a crown from tooth 16, detected and removed caries, did a build-up filling and crown preparation within 3 h. Students' feedback on a VAS questionnaire.	Students evaluated models based on real patient situations as good training possibilities. The lack of gingiva was disturbing.

RCT = Randomized Controlled Trial; CT = Controlled Trial; CS = Cohort Study; CCS = Case-Control-Study; OT = Observational Study.

3.5. Digital Radiography

Four studies dealt with diagnosing radiographic changes [79–81] or detecting positional errors on panoramic radiographs [82] (Table 5). Senior students showed a poor ability for approximal caries detection on both conventional and digital radiographs when compared to histo-pathologic analysis from sectioned teeth [80]. One study demonstrated that digital learning supported the development of students' diagnostic skills [81]. Another study showed that the accuracy of radiographic caries detection was improved by a computer-assisted learning calibration program, which provided feedback illustrating the actual tooth surface condition [79]. In one study, two digital systems for endodontic tooth length measurements were compared, and students' positive attitudes towards digital radiography were documented [83].

Table 5. Group 5: Digital Radiology ($n = 5$).

Study (Year)	Study Design	Theory/Practice	Participants	Materials and Methods	Results
Mileman et al. 2003 [79]	RCT	P	67	Investigated computer-assisted learning (CAL) calibration program to improves dental students' accuracy in dentin caries detection from bitewing radiographs; experimental ($n = 33$) group: used CAL with feedback for self-calibration control ($n = 34$) group.	CAL improved students' diagnostic performance; true positive ratio (sensitivity) for caries detection was significantly higher in test 76.3% than control with 66.9%, while false positive ratio (specificity) was similar (28.1 and 28.7%); diagnostic odds ratio was sig. higher in test (12.4) than in control (8.8).
Wenzel et al. 2004 [83]	RCT	P	31	Compared 2 digital systems (RVG-ui CCD sensor, Digora PSP plate system) for radiographic examination; after education in digital radiography one student group started with CCD, one with PSP and both completed endodontic treatment of single-rooted extracted tooth; groups switched radiography system and treated a 2nd tooth. True tooth length (TTL) and root filling length (RFL) were measured with the software and compared to manual measurement; feed-back questionnaire after each treatment.	Using CCD sensor required less time than PSP; positioning the tooth was easier with PSP plate; positive attitudes towards digital radiography; lengths measured on the digital images from both digital systems were slightly larger than true tooth lengths with no difference in ratio TTL/RFL between systems.

Table 5. *Cont.*

Study (Year)	Study Design	Theory/Practice	Participants	Materials and Methods	Results
Minston et al. 2013 [80]	CT	P	20	Investigated students' diagnostic performance on approximal caries detection with analog and digital radiographs from 46 extracted human premolars and molars, compared diagnostic accuracy; teeth were sectioned and histopathologically analyzed (gold standard)	Students ability for caries detection was poor, no difference between analog and digital radiographs.
Busanello et al. 2015 [81]	CCS	P	62	Evaluated digital learning object to improve skills in diagnosing radiographic dental changes (Visual Basic Application software); test group used the digital tool, control group: conventional imaging diagnosis course; diagnosis test after 3 weeks.	Test group performed significantly better, females were better than males.
Kratz et al. 2018 [82]	CT	P	169	Evaluated students' ability to identify positional errors (tongue position, head rotation, chin position) in panoramic radiographs of edentulous patients, students in 2nd year ($n = 84$) and 3rd–4th year ($n = 85$)	2nd year students identified significantly more positional errors than 3rd and 4th students. Students were more experienced at identifying radiographic findings compared to positional errors.

RCT = Randomized Controlled Trial; CT = Controlled Trial; CS = Cohort Study; CCS = Case-Control-Study; OT = Observational Study; CCD = Charged Couple Device; PSP = Photostimulable Phosphor.

3.6. Surveys Related to the Penetration and Acceptance of Digital Education

Six surveys evaluated students' perception and acceptance of digital technologies (Table 6) [84–89]. The more recent studies reflected that digital technologies have become established teaching tools, particularly in the field of digital radiography and microscopy, and the use of textbooks decreased; simulation training was preferred [86,87].

Table 6. Surveys related to digital education ($n = 10$).

Study (Year)	Study Design	Theory/Practice	Participants	Materials and Methods	Results
Scarfe et al. 1996 [88]	OT	T	277	Investigated the effects of instructions in intraoral digital radiology on dental students' knowledge, attitudes and beliefs; 174 from a university with formal instruction on digital dental radiography, and 103 from a university without instructions.	Students with instructions knew significantly more than students without; 93% wanted digital radiology to be included in the dental curriculum.
McCann et al. 2010 [85]	OT	T	366	Surveyed student's (dental and dental hygiene) preferences for e-teaching and learning, using an online questionnaire in 2008 related to computer experience, use and effectiveness of e-resources, preferences for various environments, need for standardization, and preferred modes of communication.	64% preferred printed text over digital and 74% wanted e-materials to supplement but not replace lectures; 71% preferred buying traditional textbooks, 11% preferred electronic versions; among e-resources virtual microscopy (69%), digital skull atlas (68%), and digital tooth atlas (64%) were reported as most effective; e-materials would enhance learning, in particular e-lectures (59%), clinical videos (54%), and podcasts (45%). E-resources should not replace interactions with faculty; students wanted lectures and clinical procedures recorded.
Jathanna et al. 2014 [84]	OT	T	186	Surveyed the perception of Indian dental students toward usefulness of digital technologies in improving dental practice, willingness to use digital and electronic technologies, perceived obstacles to use digital and electronic technologies in dental care setups, and their attitudes toward internet privacy issues.	Students indicated that digital technology increases patient satisfaction and practice efficiency, improves record quality, doctor-doctor communication, case diagnosis and treatment planning; obstacles to the wide adoption of these technologies were cost and dentists' lack of knowledge and comfort with technology.
Chatham et al. 2014 [90]	OT	T	11	Surveyed the penetration of digital technologies in UK dental schools (11/16 responded).	45% did not teach digital technologies (36% because it was not part of the curriculum, or in 95% due to the lack of technical expertise or support); half of those teaching digital technologies did so with lectures or demonstrations, the other half allowed practical involvement.

Table 6. *Cont.*

Study (Year)	Study Design	Theory/Practice	Participants	Materials and Methods	Results
Brownstein et al. 2015 [91]	OT	T	33	Surveyed the penetration of emerging dental technologies into the curricula at US dental schools (62 eligible schools were contacted); academic Deans answered 19 questions related to 12 dental topics; 19 schools had <100 students/class; 14 had >100 students.	Highest penetration was in preclinical didactic courses (62%) and lowest was in preclinical laboratory (36%); most common specific technologies were digital radiography (85%) and rotary endodontics (81%), least common were CAD/CAM denture fabrication (20%) and hard tissue lasers (24%); the bigger the class sizes (>100 students) and the older the school, the lower the incorporation of newer technologies.
Bhardwaj et al. 2015 [92]	OT	T	54	Surveyed faculties' opinion (15 dental, 42 medical faculty members in Melaka, Malaysia) toward the existing e-learning activities, and to analyze the extent of adopting and integration of e-learning into their traditional teaching methods; questionnaire with socio-demographic profile, skills and aptitude on the use of computer, knowledge and use of existing e-learning technology (e.g., MOODLE), experiences and attitudes towards e-learning, faculty opinion on novel e-learning techniques, and initiatives to be adopted for optimization of existing e-learning facilities.	65.4% of faculty was positive towards e-learning; formal training required to support e-learning that enables smooth transition of the faculty from traditional teaching into blended approach; traditional instructor centered teaching is shifting to learner centered model facilitating students to control their own learning. Popular e-learning education tools: Virtual Learning Environment systems such as WebCT™.
Ren et al. 2017 [86]	OT	T	389	Questionnaire assessed students' attitudes towards digital simulation technologies and teaching methods, how students compare digital technologies with traditional training methods; four categories: digital microscope, virtual pathology slides, digital radiography, virtual simulation training.	Most students accepted digital technologies as stimulating tool for self-learning; digital X-ray images were used to study oral radiology and preferred to conventional X-rays. Dental simulation training was most preferred technology (54.6%), 16.7% preferred digital microscopy, 15.0% virtual pathology slides, 13.7% digital x-ray images. 76% used the virtual simulation training machine to study oral clinical skills; 61% felt that the simulator would be a useful addition to current pre-clinical training; 66% felt that the simulator provided a realistic virtual environment.
Roberts et al. 2019 [87]	OT	T	282 (in 2015) 129 (in 2017)	Surveyed the use of student-managed online technologies in collaborative e-learning; comparison of web-based applications and other study methods (survey in 2015 focused on Google Doc/survey in 2017 focused on all e-learning technologies).	Significant decrease in Google Docs overall usage in 2017 (95%) compared to 2015 (99%), but significantly increased frequency of use in all courses from 36% (2015) to 71.6% (2017). The use of textbooks dropped significantly from 25% (2015) to 15% (2017). Only 4% reported that textbooks were worth the cost. 52% would not use textbooks to study even when placed at disposal. In 2017 52% spent study time with social media (Twitter or Facebook), 66% "sometimes" questioned the validity of information posted by others in collaborative documents. To collaboratively study with peers, Google Docs and personal contacts were the top choices in 2017.
Prager & Liss 2019 [2]	OT	T	54	Surveyed the extent of teaching digital modalities and use for patient care in dental schools (54 out of 76 dental schools in U.S. and Canada responded) in February 2019.	93% used CAD/CAM digital scanning, IOS was performed exclusively in 55%, extraoral model scan was used as sole technique in 8%, intra- and extraoral scanning in 37% of the schools. IOS was applied for crowns (100%), inlays/onlays (77%), implant crowns (52%), fixed partial denture (34%), complete denture (2%), but none of the schools indicated to use IOS always for crowns. 59% had a digital workflow established to deliver same-day restorations. 34% had at least 10% of faculty proficient in IOS, 66% had 10% or less.
Turkyilmaz et al. 2019 [89]	OT	T	255	Surveyed students' perception of e-learning impact on dental education, response rate of 22.6% (255 out of 1130 electronically distributed 14-question surveys to 2nd–4th year students).	48.6% preferred traditional lecture mixed with online learning, 18.4% online classes only, 18.0% traditional lecture style only; greatest impact on learning had YouTube, Bone Box, and Google. 60% spent between 1 and >4 h per day on electronic resources for academic performance. E-learning had a significant perceived effect on didactic and clinical understanding. Students observed that faculties estimated <50 years of age were more likely to incorporate e-learning into courses and more likely to use social media for communication.

RCT = Randomized Controlled Trial; CT = Controlled Trial; CS = Cohort Study; CCS = Case-Control-Study; OT = Observational Study.

Four surveys analyzed the penetration of and attitudes towards digital technologies at dental schools in the UK [90], U.S. [91], North America [2], or among the faculty staff at a dental school in Malaysia [92]. According to the most recent survey, CAD/CAM technologies were taught in most dental schools in North America (93%), while other digital modalities showed less penetration [2].

Despite a high acceptance of digital technologies in dental education by faculty [92] and students [86], it was concluded that e-resources should not replace interactions with faculty; students wanted lectures and clinical procedures recorded [85].

4. Discussion

The systematic review aimed to investigate current penetration and educational quality enhancements from digitalization in the dental curriculum. Heterogeneous study types addressing various fields of digital applications were found. While a meta-analysis was not feasible, a descriptive approach for identified publications was conducted.

Digitalization in dental education is frequently used to enhance the accessibility and exchange of documents and to facilitate the collaboration and communication among students, teachers, and administrative staff. Digitalization enables cloud-based records, evaluation, and feedback, as well as the provision of e-learning modules [23]. Students today, particularly the Millennials, expect services instantly, expect to be able to download their grades, course schedules, and other information automatically, and to be able to get assistance 24 h a day. In order to satisfy these expectations, it is necessary to promote a change of mindset of the dental faculty and provide instructors with training in e-learning and e-teaching to enable theoretical and practical knowledge transfer [85]. The coronavirus disease (Covid-19) pandemic that started in 2019 caused dental schools around the world to close, and highlighted the need for alternative channels for education (e.g., Web-based learning platforms) [93]. Scheduled webinars can provide a structure for students' theoretical learning. Additional applications of digital features include educational videos illustrating clinical exams or therapeutic steps, interactive systems, adaptive systems that monitor students' ability and adjust teaching accordingly, online collaborative tools, etc. The use of pictograms instead of scripts in educational videos facilitates a language-independent application in several countries.

Especially in the field of motor skills training, digital software tools can be used to evaluate the manual abilities of potential candidates for the dental curriculum, to analyze students' preclinical preparations, to enable self-assessment, and to enhance the quality of education. The objective and exact nature of these digital evaluations helps to improve students' visualization, provides immediate feedback, and enhances instructor evaluation and student self-evaluation and self-correction [43,94]. Students can learn to self-assess their work with self-reflection and faculty guidance in conjunction with a specially designed digital evaluation tool [48]. IOS and digital impression techniques can be included early in the dental curriculum to help familiarize students with ongoing development in the computer-assisted technologies used in oral rehabilitation [3,72].

While undergraduate students today have to be prepared for digital dentistry, they still need to acquire the knowledge of conventional treatment strategies and processes. Growing up in the digital world, they will easily adapt to digital features. Digital dentistry offers several options for an objective standardized evaluation of students' performance, which should be used for quality enhancement. It is currently a "teaching transition time", and new standards have to be defined for dental education in general. Open questions remain, such as: (i) in which phase of the dental curricula should digital technologies be introduced as the routine tool; (ii) which analog techniques can be omitted; and iii) which digital content should be taught in which disciplines?

Several studies indicated that personal instruction and feedback from faculty cannot be replaced by simulator training and feedback [39,65,85]. In this context, faculty should be aware of their responsibility in teaching young dentists, who are treating individuals with individual needs requiring empathy and an informed consent for any treatment decision. Digitalization cannot replace all educational lessons or courses, and the role-model function of faculty is important when supervising students during patient treatment in the clinical courses.

It should be emphasized that there are still no uniform standards in dental education with regard to the digital tools applied. Such standards are essential to ensure uniformity in teaching, which is particularly important for an international exchange. Society as well as dentistry is currently undergoing a digital transformation. It is necessary to clarify learning contents, to what extent conventional workflows should still be taught, and what can be done digitally. While digital tools and applications in knowledge transfer are a general challenge for undergraduate education in all disciplines, the field of dentistry with its high degree of practical training units is specifically demanding. Just because training units are designed digitally does not mean that students learn on their own. Continuous training with supervision and feed-back is still the key to good dental education. In this context, digitization is certainly a great opportunity to convey the learning content with more joy and newly awakened enthusiasm.

Following the rule, "you can only teach what you are able to perform yourself", a highly motivated faculty is needed that is willing to embrace the latest digital technologies. Besides personal motivation, the financial aspect of implementing the various digital tools and applications has to be managed at dental universities. Collaborations with industry would be helpful here. This is a classic "win–win situation"—the dental school would be equipped with the latest products and updates, and the industry would get access to the youngest target group of potential customers. In the event of such collaborations, it is vital that universities maintain their objectivity by offering a variety of products from diverse companies; otherwise, there is a risk of unduly influencing dental students and biasing them towards one particular technological option. The rapid pace of change in dental technology must also be considered. Dental technology companies are constantly introducing new products and workflows. While this provides exciting opportunities for dental research, to test and analyze those new developments, it complicates the implementation of digital workflows in dental education programs. New job descriptions are also necessary at dental schools in order to maintain the technical infrastructures required for these new technologies and to guarantee a smooth operation in clinical practice. In future, the best dental schools will be ranked according to their digital infrastructure combined with the level of innovation of the teaching faculty.

5. Conclusions

Digital tools and applications are now widespread in routine dental care. Therefore, this trend towards digitization and ongoing developments must be considered in dental curricula in order to prepare future dentists for their daily work-life. There is a need to establish generally accepted digital standards of education—at least among the different dental universities within individual countries. Digitalization offers the potential to revolutionize the entire field of dental education. More interactive and intuitive e-learning possibilities will arise that motivate students and provide a stimulating, enjoyable, and meaningful educational experience with convenient access 24 h a day.

At present, digital dental education encompasses several areas of teaching interests, including Web-based knowledge transfer and specific technologies such as digital surface mapping, dental simulator motor skills including IOS, and digital radiography. Furthermore, it is assumed that AR/VR-technology will play a dominant role in the future development of dental education.

Supplementary Materials: The following are available online at http://www.mdpi.com/1660-4601/17/9/3269/s1, Annex S1 and Annex S2.

Author Contributions: Conceptualization, Methodology, and Writing—Original Draft Preparation, N.U.Z. and T.J.; Writing—Review and Editing, N.U.Z., T.J., L.M., and H.O.; Supervision, N.U.Z. and T.J.; Project Administration, T.J. All authors have read and agreed to the published version of the manuscript.

Funding: This research received no external funding.

Conflicts of Interest: The authors declare no conflicts of interest.

References

1. Fernandez, M.A.; Nimmo, A.; Behar-Horenstein, L.S. Digital Denture Fabrication in Pre- and Postdoctoral Education: A Survey of U.S. Dental Schools. *J. Prosthodont.* **2016**, *25*, 83–90. [CrossRef] [PubMed]
2. Prager, M.C.; Liss, H. Assessment of Digital Workflow in Predoctoral Education and Patient Care in North American Dental Schools. *J. Dent. Educ.* **2019**. [CrossRef]
3. Joda, T.; Lenherr, P.; Dedem, P.; Kovaltschuk, I.; Bragger, U.; Zitzmann, N.U. Time efficiency, difficulty, and operator's preference comparing digital and conventional implant impressions: A randomized controlled trial. *Clin. Oral Implant. Res.* **2017**, *28*, 1318–1323. [CrossRef] [PubMed]
4. Joda, T.; Ferrari, M.; Bragger, U.; Zitzmann, N.U. Patient Reported Outcome Measures (PROMs) of posterior single-implant crowns using digital workflows: A randomized controlled trial with a three-year follow-up. *Clin. Oral Implant. Res.* **2018**, *29*, 954–961. [CrossRef] [PubMed]
5. Muhlemann, S.; Sandrini, G.; Ioannidis, A.; Jung, R.E.; Hammerle, C.H.F. The use of digital technologies in dental practices in Switzerland: A cross-sectional survey. *Swiss Dent. J.* **2019**, *129*, 700–707.
6. Joda, T.; Zarone, F.; Ferrari, M. The complete digital workflow in fixed prosthodontics: A systematic review. *BMC Oral Health* **2017**, *17*, 124. [CrossRef]
7. Goodacre, C.J. Digital Learning Resources for Prosthodontic Education: The Perspectives of a Long-Term Dental Educator Regarding 4 Key Factors. *J. Prosthodont.* **2018**, *27*, 791–797. [CrossRef]
8. De Boer, I.R.; Wesselink, P.R.; Vervoorn, J.M. The creation of virtual teeth with and without tooth pathology for a virtual learning environment in dental education. *Eur. J. Dent. Educ.* **2013**, *17*, 191–197. [CrossRef]
9. Joda, T.; Gallucci, G.O.; Wismeijer, D.; Zitzmann, N.U. Augmented and virtual reality in dental medicine: A systematic review. *Comput. Biol. Med.* **2019**, *108*, 93–100. [CrossRef]
10. Towers, A.; Field, J.; Stokes, C.; Maddock, S.; Martin, N. A scoping review of the use and application of virtual reality in pre-clinical dental education. *Br. Dent. J.* **2019**, *226*, 358–366. [CrossRef]
11. Moher, D.; Liberati, A.; Tetzlaff, J.; Altman, D.G.; Group, P. Preferred reporting items for systematic reviews and meta-analyses: The PRISMA statement. *Ann. Intern. Med.* **2009**, *151*, 264–269. [CrossRef]
12. Komolpis, R.; Johnson, R.A. Web-based orthodontic instruction and assessment. *J. Dent. Educ.* **2002**, *66*, 650–658. [PubMed]
13. Bains, M.; Reynolds, P.A.; McDonald, F.; Sherriff, M. Effectiveness and acceptability of face-to-face, blended and e-learning: A randomised trial of orthodontic undergraduates. *Eur. J. Dent. Educ.* **2011**, *15*, 110–117. [CrossRef] [PubMed]
14. Wright, E.F.; Hendricson, W.D. Evaluation of a 3-D interactive tooth atlas by dental students in dental anatomy and endodontics courses. *J. Dent. Educ.* **2010**, *74*, 110–122. [PubMed]
15. Mitov, G.; Dillschneider, T.; Abed, M.R.; Hohenberg, G.; Pospiech, P. Introducing and evaluating MorphoDent, a Web-based learning program in dental morphology. *J. Dent. Educ.* **2010**, *74*, 1133–1139. [PubMed]
16. Curnier, F. Teaching dentistry by means of virtual reality—The Geneva project. *Int. J. Comput. Dent.* **2010**, *13*, 251–263.
17. Kingsley, K.V.; Kingsley, K. A case study for teaching information literacy skills. *BMC Med. Educ.* **2009**, *9*, 7. [CrossRef]
18. Gonzalez, S.M.; Gadbury-Amyot, C.C. Using Twitter for Teaching and Learning in an Oral and Maxillofacial Radiology Course. *J. Dent. Educ.* **2016**, *80*, 149–155.
19. Vuchkova, J.; Maybury, T.; Farah, C.S. Digital interactive learning of oral radiographic anatomy. *Eur. J. Dent. Educ.* **2012**, *16*, e79–e87. [CrossRef]
20. Schultze-Mosgau, S.; Zielinski, T.; Lochner, J. Web-based, virtual course units as a didactic concept for medical teaching. *Med. Teach.* **2004**, *26*, 336–342. [CrossRef]
21. Qi, S.; Yan, Y.; Li, R.; Hu, J. The impact of active versus passive use of 3D technology: A study of dental students at Wuhan University, China. *J. Dent. Educ.* **2013**, *77*, 1536–1542. [PubMed]
22. Reissmann, D.R.; Sierwald, I.; Berger, F.; Heydecke, G. A model of blended learning in a preclinical course in prosthetic dentistry. *J. Dent. Educ.* **2015**, *79*, 157–165. [PubMed]
23. Alves, L.S.; de Oliveira, R.S.; Nora, A.D.; Cuozzo Lemos, L.F.; Rodrigues, J.A.; Zenkner, J.E.A. Dental Students' Performance in Detecting In Vitro Occlusal Carious Lesions Using ICDAS with E-Learning and Digital Learning Strategies. *J. Dent. Educ.* **2018**, *82*, 1077–1083. [CrossRef] [PubMed]

24. Luz, P.B.; Stringhini, C.H.; Otto, B.R.; Port, A.L.; Zaleski, V.; Oliveira, R.S.; Pereira, J.T.; Lussi, A.; Rodrigues, J.A. Performance of undergraduate dental students on ICDAS clinical caries detection after different learning strategies. *Eur. J. Dent. Educ.* **2015**, *19*, 235–241. [CrossRef] [PubMed]
25. Jackson, T.H.; Zhong, J.; Phillips, C.; Koroluk, L.D. Self-Directed Digital Learning: When Do Dental Students Study? *J. Dent. Educ.* **2018**, *82*, 373–378. [CrossRef]
26. Botelho, J.; Machado, V.; Proenca, L.; Rua, J.; Delgado, A.; Joao Mendes, J. Cloud-based collaboration and productivity tools to enhance self-perception and self-evaluation in senior dental students: A pilot study. *Eur. J. Dent. Educ.* **2019**, *23*, e53–e58. [CrossRef]
27. Boynton, J.R.; Johnson, L.A.; Nainar, S.M.; Hu, J.C. Portable digital video instruction in predoctoral education of child behavior management. *J. Dent. Educ.* **2007**, *71*, 545–549.
28. Weaver, J.M.; Lu, M.; McCloskey, K.L.; Herndon, E.S.; Tanaka, W. Digital multimedia instruction enhances teaching oral and maxillofacial suturing. *J. Calif. Dent. Assoc.* **2009**, *37*, 859–862.
29. Smith, W.; Rafeek, R.; Marchan, S.; Paryag, A. The use of video-clips as a teaching aide. *Eur. J. Dent. Educ.* **2012**, *16*, 91–96. [CrossRef]
30. Schittek Janda, M.; Mattheos, N.; Nattestad, A.; Wagner, A.; Nebel, D.; Farbom, C.; Le, D.H.; Attstrom, R. Simulation of patient encounters using a virtual patient in periodontology instruction of dental students: Design, usability, and learning effect in history-taking skills. *Eur. J. Dent. Educ.* **2004**, *8*, 111–119. [CrossRef]
31. Reynolds, P.A.; Harper, J.; Dunne, S.; Cox, M.; Myint, Y.K. Portable digital assistants (PDAs) in dentistry: Part II—Pilot study of PDA use in the dental clinic. *Br. Dent. J.* **2007**, *202*, 477–483. [CrossRef] [PubMed]
32. Pyorala, E.; Maenpaa, S.; Heinonen, L.; Folger, D.; Masalin, T.; Hervonen, H. The art of note taking with mobile devices in medical education. *BMC Med. Educ.* **2019**, *19*, 96. [CrossRef] [PubMed]
33. Mahrous, A.; Schneider, G.B.; Holloway, J.A.; Dawson, D.V. Enhancing Student Learning in Removable Partial Denture Design by Using Virtual Three-Dimensional Models Versus Traditional Two-Dimensional Drawings: A Comparative Study. *J. Prosthodont.* **2019**, *28*, 927–933. [CrossRef]
34. Callan, R.S.; Haywood, V.B.; Cooper, J.R.; Furness, A.R.; Looney, S.W. The Validity of Using E4D Compare's "% Comparison" to Assess Crown Preparations in Preclinical Dental Education. *J. Dent. Educ.* **2015**, *79*, 1445–1451. [PubMed]
35. Esser, C.; Kerschbaum, T.; Winkelmann, V.; Krage, T.; Faber, F.J. A comparison of the visual and technical assessment of preparations made by dental students. *Eur. J. Dent. Educ.* **2006**, *10*, 157–161. [CrossRef]
36. Greany, T.J.; Yassin, A.; Lewis, K.C. Developing an All-Digital Workflow for Dental Skills Assessment: Part I, Visual Inspection Exhibits Low Precision and Accuracy. *J. Dent. Educ.* **2019**, *83*, 1304–1313. [CrossRef]
37. Hamil, L.M.; Mennito, A.S.; Renne, W.G.; Vuthiganon, J. Dental students' opinions of preparation assessment with E4D compare software versus traditional methods. *J. Dent. Educ.* **2014**, *78*, 1424–1431.
38. Kateeb, E.T.; Kamal, M.S.; Kadamani, A.M.; Abu Hantash, R.O.; Abu Arqoub, M.M. Utilising an innovative digital software to grade pre-clinical crown preparation exercise. *Eur. J. Dent. Educ.* **2017**, *21*, 220–227. [CrossRef]
39. Kozarovska, A.; Larsson, C. Implementation of a digital preparation validation tool in dental skills laboratory training. *Eur. J. Dent. Educ.* **2018**, *22*, 115–121. [CrossRef]
40. Kunkel, T.C.; Engelmeier, R.L.; Shah, N.H. A comparison of crown preparation grading via PrepCheck versus grading by dental school instructors. *Int. J. Comput. Dent.* **2018**, *21*, 305–311.
41. Liu, L.; Li, J.; Yuan, S.; Wang, T.; Chu, F.; Lu, X.; Hu, J.; Wang, C.; Yan, B.; Wang, L. Evaluating the effectiveness of a preclinical practice of tooth preparation using digital training system: A randomised controlled trial. *Eur. J. Dent. Educ.* **2018**, *22*, e679–e686. [CrossRef]
42. Mays, K.A.; Crisp, H.A.; Vos, P. Utilizing CAD/CAM to Measure Total Occlusal Convergence of Preclinical Dental Students' Crown Preparations. *J. Dent. Educ.* **2016**, *80*, 100–107.
43. Miyazono, S.; Shinozaki, Y.; Sato, H.; Isshi, K.; Yamashita, J. Use of Digital Technology to Improve Objective and Reliable Assessment in Dental Student Simulation Laboratories. *J. Dent. Educ.* **2019**, *83*, 1224–1232. [CrossRef] [PubMed]
44. Park, C.F.; Sheinbaum, J.M.; Tamada, Y.; Chandiramani, R.; Lian, L.; Lee, C.; Da Silva, J.; Ishikawa-Nagai, S. Dental Students' Perceptions of Digital Assessment Software for Preclinical Tooth Preparation Exercises. *J. Dent. Educ.* **2017**, *81*, 597–603. [CrossRef] [PubMed]
45. Gratton, D.G.; Kwon, S.R.; Blanchette, D.; Aquilino, S.A. Impact of Digital Tooth Preparation Evaluation Technology on Preclinical Dental Students' Technical and Self-Evaluation Skills. *J. Dent. Educ.* **2016**, *80*, 91–99. [PubMed]

46. Gratton, D.G.; Kwon, S.R.; Blanchette, D.R.; Aquilino, S.A. Performance of two different digital evaluation systems used for assessing pre-clinical dental students' prosthodontic technical skills. *Eur. J. Dent. Educ.* **2017**, *21*, 252–260. [CrossRef] [PubMed]
47. Kwon, S.R.; Restrepo-Kennedy, N.; Dawson, D.V.; Hernandez, M.; Denehy, G.; Blanchette, D.; Gratton, D.G.; Aquilino, S.A.; Armstrong, S.R. Dental anatomy grading: Comparison between conventional visual and a novel digital assessment technique. *J. Dent. Educ.* **2014**, *78*, 1655–1662.
48. Garrett, P.H.; Faraone, K.L.; Patzelt, S.B.; Keaser, M.L. Comparison of Dental Students' Self-Directed, Faculty, and Software-Based Assessments of Dental Anatomy Wax-Ups: A Retrospective Study. *J. Dent. Educ.* **2015**, *79*, 1437–1444.
49. Mays, K.A.; Levine, E. Dental students' self-assessment of operative preparations using CAD/CAM: A preliminary analysis. *J. Dent. Educ.* **2014**, *78*, 1673–1680.
50. Sly, M.M.; Barros, J.A.; Streckfus, C.F.; Arriaga, D.M.; Patel, S.A. Grading Class I Preparations in Preclinical Dental Education: E4D Compare Software vs. the Traditional Standard. *J. Dent. Educ.* **2017**, *81*, 1457–1462. [CrossRef]
51. Lee, C.; Kobayashi, H.; Lee, S.R.; Ohyama, H. The Role of Digital 3D Scanned Models in Dental Students' Self-Assessments in Preclinical Operative Dentistry. *J. Dent. Educ.* **2018**, *82*, 399–405. [CrossRef] [PubMed]
52. Nagy, Z.A.; Simon, B.; Toth, Z.; Vag, J. Evaluating the efficiency of the Dental Teacher system as a digital preclinical teaching tool. *Eur. J. Dent. Educ.* **2018**, *22*, e619–e623. [CrossRef] [PubMed]
53. Wolgin, M.; Grabowski, S.; Elhadad, S.; Frank, W.; Kielbassa, A.M. Comparison of a prepCheck-supported self-assessment concept with conventional faculty supervision in a pre-clinical simulation environment. *Eur. J. Dent. Educ.* **2018**, *22*, e522–e529. [CrossRef] [PubMed]
54. Rees, J.S.; Jenkins, S.M.; James, T.; Dummer, P.M.; Bryant, S.; Hayes, S.J.; Oliver, S.; Stone, D.; Fenton, C. An initial evaluation of virtual reality simulation in teaching pre-clinical operative dentistry in a UK setting. *Eur. J. Prosthodont. Restor. Dent.* **2007**, *15*, 89–92.
55. Welk, A.; Maggio, M.P.; Simon, J.F.; Scarbecz, M.; Harrison, J.A.; Wicks, R.A.; Gilpatrick, R.O. Computer-assisted learning and simulation lab with 40 DentSim units. *Int. J. Comput. Dent.* **2008**, *11*, 17–40.
56. Gal, G.B.; Weiss, E.I.; Gafni, N.; Ziv, A. Preliminary assessment of faculty and student perception of a haptic virtual reality simulator for training dental manual dexterity. *J. Dent. Educ.* **2011**, *75*, 496–504.
57. Pohlenz, P.; Grobe, A.; Petersik, A.; von Sternberg, N.; Pflesser, B.; Pommert, A.; Hohne, K.H.; Tiede, U.; Springer, I.; Heiland, M. Virtual dental surgery as a new educational tool in dental school. *J. Cranio-Maxillofac. Surg.* **2010**, *38*, 560–564. [CrossRef]
58. Urbankova, A. Impact of computerized dental simulation training on preclinical operative dentistry examination scores. *J. Dent. Educ.* **2010**, *74*, 402–409.
59. Gottlieb, R.; Lanning, S.K.; Gunsolley, J.C.; Buchanan, J.A. Faculty impressions of dental students' performance with and without virtual reality simulation. *J. Dent. Educ.* **2011**, *75*, 1443–1451.
60. LeBlanc, V.R.; Urbankova, A.; Hadavi, F.; Lichtenthal, R.M. A preliminary study in using virtual reality to train dental students. *J. Dent. Educ.* **2004**, *68*, 378–383.
61. Murbay, S.; Neelakantan, P.; Chang, J.W.W.; Yeung, S. Evaluation of the introduction of a dental virtual simulator on the performance of undergraduate dental students in the pre-clinical operative dentistry course. *Eur. J. Dent. Educ.* **2019**. [CrossRef] [PubMed]
62. Kikuchi, H.; Ikeda, M.; Araki, K. Evaluation of a virtual reality simulation system for porcelain fused to metal crown preparation at Tokyo Medical and Dental University. *J. Dent. Educ.* **2013**, *77*, 782–792.
63. Ben-Gal, G.; Weiss, E.I.; Gafni, N.; Ziv, A. Testing manual dexterity using a virtual reality simulator: Reliability and validity. *Eur. J. Dent. Educ.* **2013**, *17*, 138–142. [CrossRef] [PubMed]
64. Jasinevicius, T.R.; Landers, M.; Nelson, S.; Urbankova, A. An evaluation of two dental simulation systems: Virtual reality versus contemporary non-computer-assisted. *J. Dent. Educ.* **2004**, *68*, 1151–1162. [PubMed]
65. Quinn, F.; Keogh, P.; McDonald, A.; Hussey, D. A study comparing the effectiveness of conventional training and virtual reality simulation in the skills acquisition of junior dental students. *Eur. J. Dent. Educ.* **2003**, *7*, 164–169. [CrossRef]
66. Wang, D.; Zhao, S.; Li, T.; Zhang, Y.; Wang, X. Preliminary evaluation of a virtual reality dental simulation system on drilling operation. *Biomed. Mater. Eng.* **2015**, *26* (Suppl. 1), S747–S756. [CrossRef]

67. de Boer, I.R.; Lagerweij, M.D.; Wesselink, P.R.; Vervoorn, J.M. The Effect of Variations in Force Feedback in a Virtual Reality Environment on the Performance and Satisfaction of Dental Students. *Simul. Healthc.* **2019**, *14*, 169–174. [CrossRef]
68. Schwindling, F.S.; Deisenhofer, U.K.; Porsche, M.; Rammelsberg, P.; Kappel, S.; Stober, T. Establishing CAD/CAM in Preclinical Dental Education: Evaluation of a Hands-On Module. *J. Dent. Educ.* **2015**, *79*, 1215–1221.
69. Douglas, R.D.; Hopp, C.D.; Augustin, M.A. Dental students' preferences and performance in crown design: Conventional wax-added versus CAD. *J. Dent. Educ.* **2014**, *78*, 1663–1672.
70. Wegner, K.; Michel, K.; Seelbach, P.H.; Wostmann, B. A questionnaire on the use of digital denture impressions in a preclinical setting. *Int. J. Comput. Dent.* **2017**, *20*, 177–192.
71. Schott, T.C.; Arsalan, R.; Weimer, K. Students' perspectives on the use of digital versus conventional dental impression techniques in orthodontics. *BMC Med. Educ.* **2019**, *19*, 81. [CrossRef] [PubMed]
72. Zitzmann, N.U.; Kovaltschuk, I.; Lenherr, P.; Dedem, P.; Joda, T. Dental Students' Perceptions of Digital and Conventional Impression Techniques: A Randomized Controlled Trial. *J. Dent. Educ.* **2017**, *81*, 1227–1232. [CrossRef] [PubMed]
73. Lee, S.J.; Gallucci, G.O. Digital vs. conventional implant impressions: Efficiency outcomes. *Clin. Oral Implant. Res.* **2013**, *24*, 111–115. [CrossRef]
74. Marti, A.M.; Harris, B.T.; Metz, M.J.; Morton, D.; Scarfe, W.C.; Metz, C.J.; Lin, W.S. Comparison of digital scanning and polyvinyl siloxane impression techniques by dental students: Instructional efficiency and attitudes towards technology. *Eur. J. Dent. Educ.* **2017**, *21*, 200–205. [CrossRef] [PubMed]
75. Kattadiyil, M.T.; Jekki, R.; Goodacre, C.J.; Baba, N.Z. Comparison of treatment outcomes in digital and conventional complete removable dental prosthesis fabrications in a predoctoral setting. *J. Prosthet. Dent.* **2015**, *114*, 818–825. [CrossRef]
76. Murrell, M.; Marchini, L.; Blanchette, D.; Ashida, S. Intraoral Camera Use in a Dental School Clinic: Evaluations by Faculty, Students, and Patients. *J. Dent. Educ.* **2019**, *83*, 1339–1344. [CrossRef]
77. Soares, P.V.; de Almeida Milito, G.; Pereira, F.A.; Reis, B.R.; Soares, C.J.; de Sousa Menezes, M.; de Freitas Santos-Filho, P.C. Rapid prototyping and 3D-virtual models for operative dentistry education in Brazil. *J. Dent. Educ.* **2013**, *77*, 358–363.
78. Kroger, E.; Dekiff, M.; Dirksen, D. 3D printed simulation models based on real patient situations for hands-on practice. *Eur. J. Dent. Educ.* **2017**, *21*, e119–e125. [CrossRef]
79. Mileman, P.A.; van den Hout, W.B.; Sanderink, G.C. Randomized controlled trial of a computer-assisted learning program to improve caries detection from bitewing radiographs. *Dentomaxillofac. Radiol.* **2003**, *32*, 116–123. [CrossRef]
80. Minston, W.; Li, G.; Wennberg, R.; Nasstrom, K.; Shi, X.Q. Comparison of diagnostic performance on approximal caries detection among Swedish and Chinese senior dental students using analogue and digital radiographs. *Swed. Dent. J.* **2013**, *37*, 79–85.
81. Busanello, F.H.; da Silveira, P.F.; Liedke, G.S.; Arus, N.A.; Vizzotto, M.B.; Silveira, H.E.; Silveira, H.L. Evaluation of a digital learning object (DLO) to support the learning process in radiographic dental diagnosis. *Eur. J. Dent. Educ.* **2015**, *19*, 222–228. [CrossRef]
82. Kratz, R.J.; Nguyen, C.T.; Walton, J.N.; MacDonald, D. Dental Students' Interpretations of Digital Panoramic Radiographs on Completely Edentate Patients. *J. Dent. Educ.* **2018**, *82*, 313–321. [CrossRef]
83. Wenzel, A.; Kirkevang, L.L. Students' attitudes to digital radiography and measurement accuracy of two digital systems in connection with root canal treatment. *Eur. J. Dent. Educ.* **2004**, *8*, 167–171. [CrossRef]
84. Jathanna, V.R.; Jathanna, R.V.; Jathanna, R. The awareness and attitudes of students of one Indian dental school toward information technology and its use to improve patient care. *Educ. Health (Abingdon)* **2014**, *27*, 293–296. [CrossRef] [PubMed]
85. McCann, A.L.; Schneiderman, E.D.; Hinton, R.J. E-teaching and learning preferences of dental and dental hygiene students. *J. Dent. Educ.* **2010**, *74*, 65–78. [PubMed]
86. Ren, Q.; Wang, Y.; Zheng, Q.; Ye, L.; Zhou, X.D.; Zhang, L.L. Survey of student attitudes towards digital simulation technologies at a dental school in China. *Eur. J. Dent. Educ.* **2017**, *21*, 180–186. [CrossRef] [PubMed]
87. Roberts, B.S.; Roberts, E.P.; Reynolds, S.; Stein, A.F. Dental Students' Use of Student-Managed Google Docs and Other Technologies in Collaborative Learning. *J. Dent. Educ.* **2019**, *83*, 437–444. [CrossRef] [PubMed]

88. Scarfe, W.C.; Potter, B.J.; Farman, A.G. Effects of instruction on the knowledge, attitudes and beliefs of dental students towards digital radiography. *Dentomaxillofac. Radiol.* **1996**, *25*, 103–108. [CrossRef]
89. Turkyilmaz, I.; Hariri, N.H.; Jahangiri, L. Student's Perception of the Impact of E-learning on Dental Education. *J. Contemp. Dent. Pract.* **2019**, *20*, 616–621. [CrossRef]
90. Chatham, C.; Spencer, M.H.; Wood, D.J.; Johnson, A. The introduction of digital dental technology into BDS curricula. *Br. Dent. J.* **2014**, *217*, 639–642. [CrossRef]
91. Brownstein, S.A.; Murad, A.; Hunt, R.J. Implementation of new technologies in U.S. dental school curricula. *J. Dent. Educ.* **2015**, *79*, 259–264.
92. Bhardwaj, A.; Nagandla, K.; Swe, K.M.; Abas, A.B. Academic Staff Perspectives Towards Adoption of E-learning at Melaka Manipal Medical College: Has E-learning Redefined our Teaching Model? *Kathmandu Univ. Med. J. (KUMJ)* **2015**, *13*, 12–18. [CrossRef]
93. Meng, L.; Hua, F.; Bian, Z. Coronavirus Disease 2019 (COVID-19): Emerging and Future Challenges for Dental and Oral Medicine. *J. Dent. Res.* **2020**. [CrossRef]
94. Greany, T.J.; Yassin, A.; Lewis, K.C. Developing an All-Digital Workflow for Dental Skills Assessment: Part II, Surface Analysis, Benchmarking, and Grading. *J. Dent. Educ.* **2019**, *83*, 1314–1322. [CrossRef]

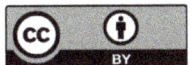

© 2020 by the authors. Licensee MDPI, Basel, Switzerland. This article is an open access article distributed under the terms and conditions of the Creative Commons Attribution (CC BY) license (http://creativecommons.org/licenses/by/4.0/).

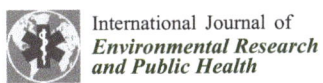 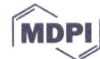

Article

Dental Practice Integration Into Primary Care: A Microsimulation of Financial Implications for Practices

Sung Eun Choi [1,*], Lisa Simon [2,3], Jane R. Barrow [2], Nathan Palmer [4], Sanjay Basu [5,6,7] and Russell S. Phillips [5]

1. Department of Oral Health Policy and Epidemiology, Harvard School of Dental Medicine, Boston, MA 02115, USA
2. Office of Global and Community Health, Harvard School of Dental Medicine, Boston, MA 02115, USA; Lisa_Simon@hms.harvard.edu (L.S.); Jane_Barrow@hsdm.harvard.edu (J.R.B)
3. Harvard Medical School, Boston, MA 02115, USA
4. Department of Biomedical Informatics, Harvard Medical School, Boston, MA 02115, USA; Nathan_Palmer@hms.harvard.edu
5. Center for Primary Care, Harvard Medical School, Boston, MA 02115, USA; Sanjay_Basu@hms.harvard.edu (S.B.); Russell_Phillips@hms.harvard.edu (R.S.P.)
6. Research and Analytics, Collective Health, San Francisco, CA 94107, USA
7. School of Public Health, Imperial College London, London SW7 2BU, UK
* Correspondence: Sung_Choi@hsdm.harvard.edu; Tel.: +1-617-432-5691

Received: 24 February 2020; Accepted: 22 March 2020; Published: 24 March 2020

Abstract: Given the widespread lack of access to dental care for many vulnerable Americans, there is a growing realization that integrating dental and primary care may provide comprehensive care. We sought to model the financial impact of integrating dental care provision into a primary care practice. A microsimulation model was used to estimate changes in net revenue per practice by simulating patient visits to a primary dental practice within primary care practices, utilizing national survey and un-identified claims data from a nationwide health insurance plan. The impact of potential changes in utilization rates and payer distributions and hiring additional staff was also evaluated. When dental care services were provided in the primary care setting, annual net revenue changes per practice were −$92,053 (95% CI: −93,054, −91,052) in the first year and $104,626 (95% CI: 103,315, 105,316) in subsequent years. Net revenue per annum after the first year of integration remained positive as long as the overall utilization rates decreased by less than 25%. In settings with a high proportion of publicly insured patients, the net revenue change decreased but was still positive. Integrating primary dental and primary care providers would be financially viable, but this viability depends on demands of dental utilization and payer distributions.

Keywords: integrated care; medical–dental integration; simulation model; dental research

1. Introduction

Dentistry has traditionally remained a separate discipline from other areas of medicine in the U.S. [1], and this artificial division does not foster comprehensive and high-quality care. Evidence shows that oral health complications, such as inflammation and infections that begin in the mouth, can lead to major health complications (e.g., dental abscess) [2]. Furthermore, a growing body of research has identified a potential connection between oral health and other chronic conditions, such as diabetes and cardiovascular diseases [3–5]. The National Academy of Medicine (an American nonprofit, non-governmental organization providing expert advice on issues relating to health, medicine, and health policy) has proposed integrating oral health into primary care as a way to expand access to recommended treatments and promote better health overall [6,7]. Despite recent studies suggesting that integration of dental care may benefit patients or reduce healthcare costs [8], financing and delivery of dental care remains disconnected from other health services, even among Accountable Care Organizations (ACOs), a network of coordinated healthcare practitioners in the U.S. that shares financial and medical responsibility for providing coordinated care to patients in the hopes of improving overall population health. Integration of dental care may present an opportunity for improved accountability for total health. However, there is little financial incentive and considerable financial uncertainties for ACOs to facilitate access to these services [6,9,10].

A number of organizations have initiated efforts to adopt integrated dental–medical care. One form of these efforts is integration in a co-located setting where provision of primary dental services is within and a part of primary care or vice versa. Co-location of medical and dental services is not a new concept; Federally Qualified Health Centers across the country have offered medical and dental facilities in the same building for decades, but often, electronic health records (EHRs) lack interoperability. A more innovative co-located model would allow communication across disciplines and sharing of patient information and EHRs, which provides an opportunity for the providers to "close the loop" on care gaps for patients beyond just providing care [11,12]. This approach facilitates timely delivery of diagnostic, preventive, and treatment services to improve patient health and reduce inefficiency in care delivery, allowing easier bidirectional referrals and quicker access for medical patients with acute oral health situations (and for dental patients with potential medical issues) [3–5,13].

Currently there are co-located facilities developing in the U.S., and pilot studies are being conducted in these settings [14]. A number of integrated care projects have had promising results, including the Colorado Medical Dental Integration Project [15,16]. One of the demonstration projects, the University of California, Los Angeles (UCLA)-First 5 LA Project, showed increased access to dental care by 85%, with the majority of services in diagnostic and preventive care [17]. While these demonstration projects are effective in assessing changes in dental care access rates and identifying logistical barriers, a key gap in knowledge is the economic viability of the delivery of such services by primary care practices constrained by financial realities. In this study, we estimated the cost and revenue implications to primary care practices of embedding a dental practice to integrate primary dental and primary medical care.

2. Materials and Methods

2.1. Study Design

We estimated costs and revenues for an integrated medical and dental practice using a microsimulation model (Figure 1), an approach often used to evaluate the effects of hypothetical interventions before they are implemented in the real world [8,18]. We simulated a representative sample of 10,000 integrated practices (dental practice embedded within the primary care practice providing dental services provided by a general dentist and dental hygienist, with supporting dental assistants), per International Society for Pharmacoeconomics and Outcomes Research (ISPOR) guidelines [19]. For each of the simulated practices, we assigned a number of simulated patient visits, then for each visit, an insurance type and indicator variables for receiving certain types of procedures were assigned, matching the overall distribution of procedure utilization rates by insurance type.

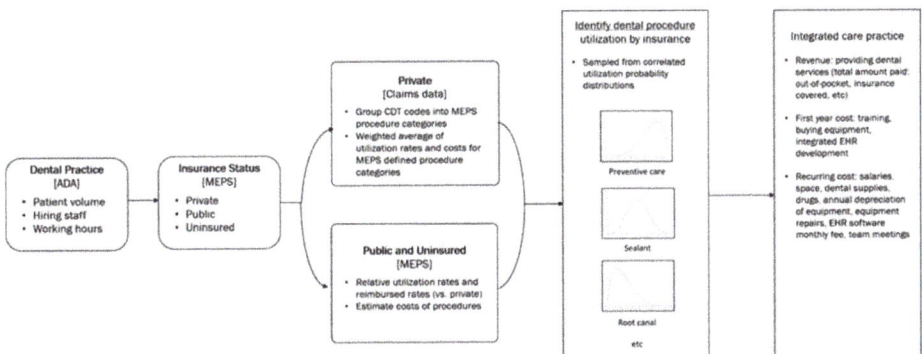

Figure 1. Simulation model flow diagram [data sources]. ADA = American Dental Association; MEPS = Medical Expenditure Panel Survey; CDT = Code on Dental Procedures and Nomenclature.

The simulation model was re-run 10,000 times while repeatedly Monte Carlo sampling from the probability distributions around the patient volume, utilization, cost, and expense data points shown in Table 1 to compute the mean and 95% credible intervals [20]. This process also accounted for the correlation among procedure utilization rates by insurance type to capture the common co-occurrence of procedures. Simulations were performed in R (v. 3.3.2, The R Foundation for Statistical Computing, Vienna, Austria). This study was reviewed by the institutional review board of the Harvard Medical School and determined to be "not-human subjects research" since the data are publicly available and de-identified.

Table 1. Input data for the dental care integration model. Data are expressed as mean (SD).

Parameters	Value	Source
Practice/patient characteristics		
Number of patient visits per dentist (including hygienist appointment) per year	3415 (347)	ADA HPI [21]
Number of patient visits per dentist (excluding hygienist appointment) per year	1831 (127)	ADA HPI [21]
Number of patient visits per hour	2.3	ADA HPI [21]
Number of hours spent on patient visits per day	6.1	ADA HPI [21]
Health insurance payer distribution of overall population (proportion with dental insurance in each group)		MEPS [22]
Private	0.66 (0.01) [0.69 (0.01)]	
Public	0.25 (0.01) [0.02 (0.01)]	
Uninsured	0.08 (0.01) [0.04 (0.01)]	

Table 1. *Cont.*

Parameters	Value	Source
Dental insurance payer distribution		MEPS [22]
Private	0.52 (0.05)	
Public	0.19 (0.03)	
Uninsured	0.29 (0.01)	
Utilization rates		
CDT procedure level utilization rate (privately insured)	Supplementary Table S1	Aetna Warehouse
Relative scales of utilization rates (public and uninsured)	Supplementary Table S1	MEPS [22]
Costs of dental procedures		
CDT procedure level costs (privately insured)	Supplementary Table S2	Aetna Warehouse
Reimbursement rates relative to private insurance	Supplementary Table S3	MEPS [22]
Expenses		
Dentist salary	152,210 (20,830)	ADA HPI [21]
Hygienist	74,070 (12,680)	Bureau of Labor Statistics [23]
Chairside assistant	37,630 (6870)	Bureau of Labor Statistics [23]
Primary care physician (hourly)	$98 (7)	MGMA [24]
Medical Assistant (hourly)	$15.1(2)	Bureau of Labor Statistics [23]
Recurring costs		
Clinical space	$1014 (290)	MGMA [24]
Dental supplies	6.4% of gross billing	ADA [25]
Drugs	0.3% of gross billing	ADA [25]
Dental lab charges	6.4% of gross billing	ADA [25]
Repairs of dental equipment	0.7% of gross billing	ADA [25]
Annual depreciation cost on dental equipment	2.2% of gross billing	ADA [25]
EHR software monthly fee	$135 (25)	Delta Dental [26]
Transition Costs (applied to the first year)		
Equipment, computers, software	$195,000 (2000)	ADA [27]
Integrated EHR development	$5000	Delta Dental [26]
Planning, coordination, informatics and workflow revision, and quality improvement during setup period	$1411 (73)	Prior pilot projects in other disciplines [28,29]

ADA = American Dental Association; HPI = Health Policy Institute; MGMA = Medical Group Management Association; EHR = electronic health records.

2.2. Model Assumption

We first estimated the patient volume that needs to be maintained at the integrated settings. On average, full-time equivalent (FTE) general dental practitioners experience 14.6 patient visits per day including dental hygienist visits [21]. An FTE primary care physician sees 19.7 patients per day on average [30]. In our model, we assumed that the minimum patient volume at the integrated settings is at least 15 patients per day, the supply of dentists remains above 61 dentists per 100,000 population with 5 primary care physicians to 1 general dental practitioner per setting. Then, we identified dental procedures that could be routinely offered by general dentists using the Code on Dental Procedures and Nomenclature (CDT Code) [31]. The final set of procedures offered in the primary care setting was determined based on the list of dental procedures covered by Adult Medicaid dental benefits in Maryland and by expert opinions from more than two general dentists to determine a conservative set of procedures (Supplementary Table S4) [32]. This final set of procedures does not include procedures that involve cost-prohibitive dental equipment for a small general dental practice, such as a Panorex machine, or are primarily billed by dentist specialists, such as orthodontic services.

2.3. Data Sources

Data sources and input data for the model are detailed in Table 1. We obtained the annual patient volume and transition costs from American Dental Association (ADA) Survey of Dental Practice [21,33]. We then subcategorized dental visits for each procedure type among patients by dental insurance type: private, public, and self-pay/uninsured based on Medical Expenditure Panel Survey (MEPS) data (for dental practices; $N = 30.5$ million) (Figure 1) [22].

We obtained the utilization rates and costs for each procedure among a privately insured population using un-identifiable member claims data from Aetna and estimated utilization rates and cost (reimbursed rates and payer distribution) among publicly insured and uninsured populations by extrapolating from MEPS (Supplementary Tables S2 and S3 and Supplementary Figure S1) [22]. Because MEPS data do not provide procedure-level utilization rates, we grouped CDT procedure codes into the procedure categories used in MEPS (Supplementary Table S4). These estimates were used to capture varying utilization and reimbursement rates by insurance status across the U.S.

2.4. Cost and Revenue Estimates from Dental–Medical Integration

We computed the cost of the embedded dental practice using procedure utilization rates and associated costs (shown in Table 1). The transition costs included the costs related to training staff and the time necessary for planning, coordination, informatics and workflow revision, and quality improvement, and start-up equipment purchase, and interoperable EHR software expenses (EHR software development cost for the first year and monthly lease fees for the subsequent years) [26]. Recurring costs included salaries for a general dental practitioner (1 full-time equivalent (FTE)), dental hygienists (1.4 FTE), and chairside assistants (1.5 FTE), and the costs associated with delivering dental services, such as dental supplies and drugs. These estimates were calculated from the fact that average general dental practitioners hire dental hygienists and chairside assistants 77.5% and 86.3% of the time, and average numbers of dental hygienists and chairside assistants per dentist among those who employ these staff are 1.8 and 1.7, respectively [34].

2.5. Primary and Secondary Outcome Metrics

The primary outcome was changes in net revenue per integrated practice per year. We computed the main outcome metric as the total reimbursements for dental services minus the total cost of service provision. Our secondary outcome metrics included (1) costs of dental service integration and (2) gross revenues for dental service integration. The primary and secondary outcomes were computed per annum for both the first and subsequent years.

2.6. Sensitivity Analyses

In an integrated setting, an increase in dental service utilization is expected due to theoretically easier access to dental care. Moreover, with recent findings on association between periodontal diseases and chronic conditions, a number of insurance companies have started offering 100% coverage for nonsurgical periodontal treatment to those with chronic conditions, such as diabetes, cardiovascular diseases, rheumatoid arthritis, and HIV/AIDS, which may increase utilization of periodontal treatment services [35–37]. The average hours per day a general dental practitioner spends in the dental office is 6.3, and 26.5% of surveyed general dentists perceived their workload to be "not busy enough" [38]. In order to estimate expected changes in net revenue from changes in utilization rates, we simulated potential increases or decreases in utilization rates in all procedure types from 50% (7 patients/day) to 120% (17 patients/day, dental practitioners spending time in the dental office for a maximum 7.6 hours per day) of baseline values.

Next, based on findings from one of the demonstration projects [17], we assessed how increases in preventive care utilization (radiographs, prophylaxis, fluoride varnish application, and sealant placement) would result in changes in net revenue. Because preventive care can be performed by hygienists, we simulated changes in net revenue from employing an additional hygienist to accommodate potential increases in preventive dental care. The number of patients a dental hygienist could accept was capped at the current average number of hygienist appointments at general dental practices nationwide [38]. We evaluated the impact of varying rates of increase in preventive care utilization on total net revenue with an additional dental hygienist.

Lastly, we simulated different payer distributions across the patient visits. In the base-case scenario, we used the national average payer distribution for medical and dental practices; 66% private, 25% public, 8 % uninsured for medical, and 52% private, 19% public, and 29% uninsured for dental practices (in dental practices, we did not include Medicare as public as dental benefits are not covered under Medicare with the exception of select Medicare Advantage plans). In this sensitivity analysis, we evaluated the impact of different patient payer distributions in certain settings. Community Health Centers (CHCs) serve a higher percentage of publicly insured or uninsured patients than the national average: 17% private, 59% public (49% Medicaid), and 24% uninsured [39]. In order to account for the fact that most patients seen by the dentist will come from the primary care practice after integration, we simulated average payer distribution at primary care practices: 45% private, 48 % public (17% Medicaid), and 7% uninsured [40]. In these scenarios, we assumed that same proportions of privately insured and Medicare patients have private dental insurance as in the base case, and calculated estimated dental insurance payer distributions for each setting.

3. Results

3.1. Base-Case Analyses

Among the fifteen procedure types that were determined to be routinely delivered by general dental practitioners, diagnostic examination and cleaning (prophylaxis) had the highest utilization rates, followed by radiographs (Supplementary Figure S2). The privately insured population visited dental practices for routine check-ups and cleanings at a higher rate than publicly insured or uninsured populations. While 62.2% (95% CI: 61.0, 63.3) of the total dental visits in a given year were for examinations in the privately insured population, publicly insured and uninsured populations visited a dental practice for examinations 57.6% (95% CI: 55.6, 59.5) and 53% (95% CI: 48.2, 58.3) of the time, respectively. However, the rate of tooth extraction was more than twice as high among publicly insured and uninsured patients, which might be due to less-frequent routine dental visits. Uninsured patients visited a dental practice for tooth extraction 21.6% (95% CI: 19.6, 23.7) of the time, whereas privately and publicly insured patients visited a dental practice for tooth extraction 5.8% (95% CI: 5.6, 6.0) and 14.4% (95% CI: 13.8, 15.0) of the time, respectively.

When dental services by a general dental practitioner were offered in the simulated integrated care setting, the primary outcome of net revenue was positive after the first year of integration. Due to transition costs and start-up expenses, the net revenue in the first year of integration was negative, -$92,053 (95% CI: −93,054, −91,052) (Table 2). After the first year, annual net revenue for the subsequent years was $104,316 (95% CI: 103,315, 105,316) per practice after the first year, assuming the same utilization rates as existing patients who completed dental visits.

Table 2. Costs and revenues from medical–dental integration, per practice per year.

	Cost, Year 1 (USD)	Cost, after Year 1 (USD)	Gross Revenue (USD)	Net Revenue, Year 1 (USD)	Net Revenue, After Year 1 (USD)
Base case	585,927 (585,335, 586,519)	389,514 (388,923, 390,104)	493,830 (492,831, 494,828)	−92,053 (−93,054, −91,052)	104,316 (103,315, 105,316)
Overall utilization (patient visit volume) change					
50%	546,758 (546,184, 547,331)	350,372 (349,799, 350,944)	247,654 (247,148, 248,160)	−299,227 (−299,929, −298,526)	−102,717 (−103,416, −102,019)
60%	554,582 (554,006, 555,158)	358,180 (357,604, 358,755)	296,759 (296,157, 297,362)	−257,842 (−258,595, −257,089)	−61,420 (−62,170, −60,669)
70%	562,408 (562,408, 561,829)	366,018 (365,439, 366,596)	346,057 (345,354, 346,760)	−216,448 (−217,256, −215,639)	−19,960 (−20,768, −19,152)
80%	570,238 (569,655, 570,821)	373,822 (373,240, 374,404)	395,141 (394,341, 395,940)	−175,034 (−175,904, −174,164)	21,318 (20,450, 22,186)
90%	578,076 (577,489, 578,663)	381,689 (381,103, 382,275)	444,617 (443,719, 445,516)	−133,575 (−134,507, −132,644)	62,928 (61,994, 63,862)
110%	593,784 (593,188, 594,381)	397,350 (396,777, 397,966)	543,252 (542,160, 544,344)	−50,490 (−51,557, −49,421)	145,880 (144,812, 146,948)
120%	601,601 (601,000, 602,202)	405,067 (404,582, 405,782)	592,374 (591,183, 593,564)	−9145 (−10,287, −8004)	187,191 (186,052, 188,330)
Preventive service utilization change with additional dental hygienist					
50% increase	673,080 (672,304, 673,857)	476,603 (475,843, 477,363)	576,377 (575,362, 577,391)	−96,703 (−97,787, −95,620)	99,774 (98,657, 100,889)
60% increase	675,706 (674,927, 676,484)	479,228 (478,469, 479,988)	592,887 (591,868, 593,907)	−82,818 (−83,897, −81,738)	113,659 (112,539, 114,778)
70% increase	678,331 (677,550, 679,112)	481,854 (481,094, 482,613)	609,399 (608,373, 610,425)	−68,932 (−70,008, −67,856)	127,545 (126,421, 128,669)
80% increase	680,955 (680,171, 681,738)	484,477 (483,717, 485,237)	625,899 (624,868, 626,931)	−55,055 (−56,127, −53,982)	141,422 (140,294, 142,550)
90% increase	683,580 (682,795, 684,366)	487,103 (486,343, 487,863)	642,413 (64,1374, 643,452)	−41,167 (−42,236, −40,097)	155,310 (154,178, 156,442)
100% increase(full capacity)	686,208 (685,420, 686,995)	489,730 (488,970, 490,491)	658,939 (657,894, 659,985)	−27,268 (−28,335, −26,201)	169,208 (168,071, 170,345)

The total gross revenue from dental practices was $493,830 (95% CI: 492,831, 494,828). The highest-revenue-generating procedure type was cleanings, with a gross revenue of $130,350 (95% CI: 130,088, 130,612), followed by diagnostic examinations and extractions, with gross annual revenues of $80,910 (95% CI: 80,747, 81,072) and $53,693 (95% CI: 53,574, 53,811), respectively (Figure 2). The least-revenue-generating procedure type was repair, such as repairing or rebasing dentures, resulting in gross annual revenue of $512 (95% CI: 508, 518).

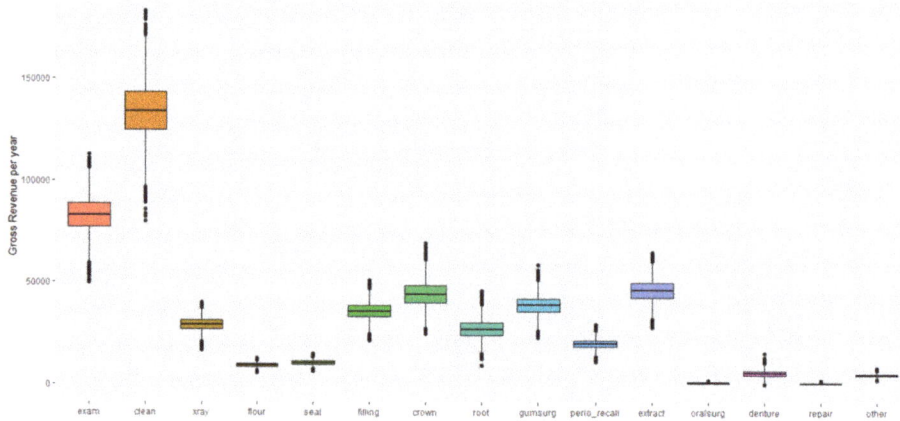

Figure 2. Gross revenue by procedure type, showing the minimum (lower whisker), maximum (upper whisker), median (center of the box), lower quartile (bottom of box), and upper quartile (top of box) values. Exam = diagnostic; clean: prophylaxis; X-ray = radiographic image; flour = fluoride; seal = sealant; root = root canal; gumsurg = periodontal scaling, root planning or gum; extract = extraction/ tooth pulled; repair = repair of bridges/dentures or relining.

3.2. Sensitivity Analyses

When overall utilization rates varied from half to twice their baseline values, net revenue per annum after the first year of integration remained positive as long as the overall utilization rates decreased by less than 25% (Table 2). Because of a greater number of adults visiting a physician annually than a dental practitioner and increased rates of enhanced dental benefits among patients with chronic conditions who are more likely to have more frequent medical visits, we expect that medical–dental integration would increase access to and utilization of dental care. When the modeled utilization rates were increased by 20%, net revenue per annum was $187,191 (95% CI: 186,052, 188,330).

Next, we evaluated the impact of hiring an additional dental hygienist to perform four types of procedures (radiographs, prophylaxis, fluoride varnish application, and sealant placement) to accommodate potential increases in preventive dental care with integration. When preventive care utilization increased by more than 53%, hiring an additional full-time dental hygienist resulted in a higher net revenue. If a full-time dental hygienist is hired and works at full capacity (performing diagnostic and preventive procedures at approximately the same rates as the average dental hygienist currently seeing patients in the U.S.), the expected net revenue was $169,208 (95% CI: 168,071, 170,345), which was a 62.2% increase from before employing the additional dental hygienist (Table 2).

When we simulated payer distributions at a CHC with a high proportion of publicly insured, the expected net revenue was $70,099 (95% CI: 69,136, 71,061), $34,217 lower than the net revenue from the base-case scenario, due primarily to lower reimbursement rates from public payers and the types of dental procedures these patients receive (Figure 3 and Supplementary Table S5). In the average primary care provider setting, the net revenue was $108,764 (95% CI: 107,744, 109,783), which was $4448 higher than the net revenue from the base-case scenario.

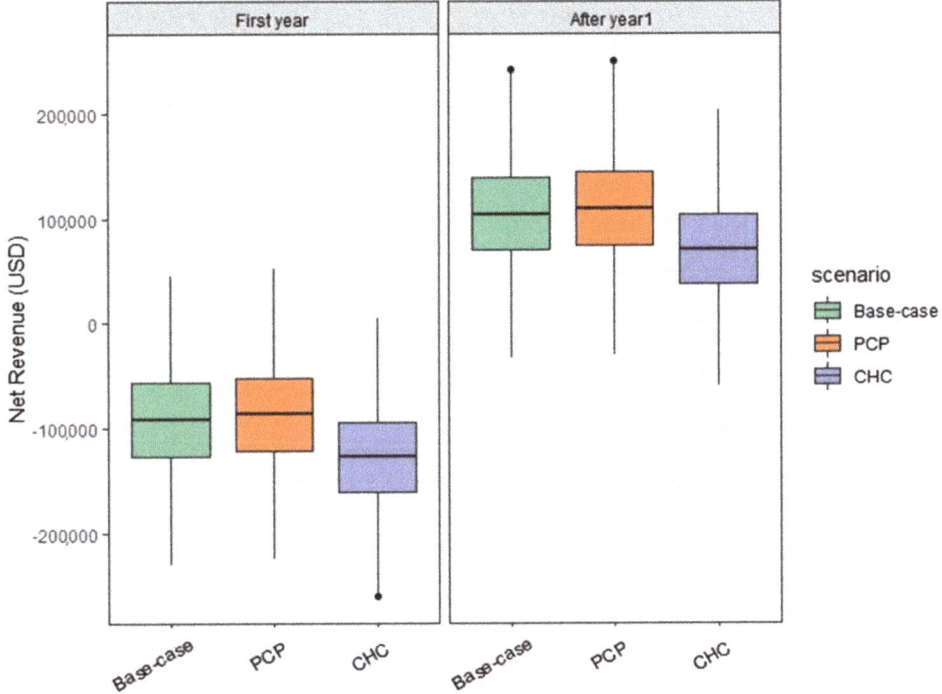

Figure 3. Impact of different payer distributions, showing the minimum (lower whisker), maximum (upper whisker), median (center of the box), lower quartile (bottom of box), and upper quartile (top of box) values. Base case = national average; PCP = primary care practice; CHC = community health center.

4. Discussion

With increased interest in the potential for integrated medical–dental care, our study evaluated the financial viability of primary integrated services—primary medicine and primary dentistry—to achieve whole-person care. We found that the net revenue changes after the first year of integration would remain positive when the integrated care could maintain at least 75% of current patient volume and the payer distribution. Serving a high proportion of patients covered by public dental insurance would result in a lower net revenue due to lower reimbursement rates. With the potential increase in utilization of basic preventive services due to integration, employing an additional hygienist to accommodate increased demand would increase the net revenue up to 62% if the hygienist worked at full capacity.

A key obstacle to successful integration of medical and dental service provision has been the substantial infrastructural investments required, such as interoperable EHRs, shared or commonly managed facilities, and a multidisciplinary workforce. While an interoperable EHR promotes well-informed care and treatment planning as well as coordination of the scheduling and billing of patient visits, it is relatively new concept and involves technical hurdles [41]. In our study, we implemented a monthly leased software option, a reasonably integrated option; however, it could be home grown with greater financial investment. For this and other reasons, the integration of medical and dental services can be a highly resource-intensive model to implement.

Our results suggest that facilities would experience negative net revenue from implementation in the first year; however, the net revenue for successful implementation would remain positive. While our study was limited to evaluating the financial viability of the integrated care, the expected benefits from this integration may extend beyond positive revenue. Integrated care facilitates timely delivery of diagnostic, preventive, and treatment services to improve patient health and reduce inefficiency in care delivery. Integrated care with dental, psychiatric, and allied health service has been also supported in other countries [42], and due to significant overlap in training between dental and medical students in many European countries, it is practically viable outside the U.S. [43]. Based on recent findings on the association between oral health status and chronic conditions [3–5] and potential cost savings from co-management of these diseases [44,45], integrated medical–dental practice could be expected to improve health outcomes of the population and result in cost savings in the overall healthcare expenditures in the U.S.

Our analysis has limitations inherent to simulation modeling based on secondary data sources. First, we simulated the utilization and cost of dental services at procedure level based on claims data from a mostly privately insured population. Although we extrapolated from nationally representative survey data to make projections about publicly insured and uninsured populations, some information loss is to be expected by grouping a number of procedure codes into different categories. An additional logical step for future research is to gain access to claims data from publicly insured populations, such as Center for Medicare and Medicaid Services (CMS) data, to identify whether incorporating procedure-level data in this population would alter the findings of our study [46]. Furthermore, we lacked sufficiently rigorous data to expand our model to incorporate regional variation in service utilization and payer distribution, such as urban vs. rural or by state. Dentist supply, dental care demand, and payer distributions vary a lot across geographic location. While our study results are based on national averages, medical–dental integration would likely yield higher revenue in one setting than the in other. In the absence of robust data about how much patient volume would change in terms of dental service need, we did not make any assumptions about the trends in dental utilization or payer distribution of the population over time. Moreover, we assumed that only a subset of dental procedures would be performed by general dental practitioners at an integrated setting under a fee-for-service scenario, and specialty services would be referred out. However, it may not be applicable to CHC where it accepts encounter-based payment, and there is a possibility that some CHCs may provide specialty services that are not covered, which would alter the financial impact of the integrated care practice. Finally, the proprietary nature of the ADA data used here is a limitation for broad usage; the potential availability of other practice cost registries or data from a strong medical–dental integrated practice may eventually lead to the wider availability of financial data for practice planning, and it remains as an area for future research.

5. Conclusions

Our findings suggest that medical–dental integration is financially viable. Given that more adults visit a physician than a dentist annually and that in some case enhanced dental benefits are being offered to patients with chronic conditions, medical–dental integration could improve patient health and reduce inefficiency in care delivery. Furthermore, it has potential value to provide comprehensive whole-person care through bidirectional referrals and sharing patient information, which would provide a critical opportunity to bridge the gap between dentistry and medicine.

Supplementary Materials: The following are available online at http://www.mdpi.com/1660-4601/17/6/2154/s1, Table S1: Utilization rates by procedure type and by insurance, Table S2: Costs by dental procedure types (commercial insurance), Table S3: Reimbursed rates by insurance status, Table S4: Procedure codes offered by general dentist and MEPS dental practice category matching, Table S5: Sensitivity analysis results—different payer distributions, Figure S1: Payment source distribution by insurance status, Figure S2: Utilization rates by procedure and insurance types

Author Contributions: S.E.C.: study conception and design, statistical analysis, acquisition of data, analysis and interpretation of data, drafting of the manuscript, and critical revision of the manuscript; N.P.: acquisition of data and critical revision of the manuscript; J.R.B.: study conception and design, acquisition of data, and critical revision of the manuscript; L.S., S.B., and R.S.P.: study conception and design and critical revision of the manuscript. All authors have read and agreed to the published version of the manuscript.

Funding: Research reported in this publication was supported by the Harvard School of Dental Medicine Initiative to Integrate Oral Health and Medicine. The content is solely the responsibility of the authors and does not necessarily represent the official views of Harvard School of Dental Medicine.

Conflicts of Interest: The authors declare no conflict of interest.

References

1. Simon, L. Overcoming Historical Separation between Oral and General Health Care: Interprofessional Collaboration for Promoting Health Equity. *AMA J. Ethics* **2016**, *18*, 941–949. [CrossRef] [PubMed]
2. Mayo Clinic. Oral Health: A Window to Your Overall Health. Available online: https://www.mayoclinic.org/healthy-lifestyle/adult-health/in-depth/dental/art-20047475 (accessed on 31 March 2019).
3. Dietrich, T.; Webb, I.; Stenhouse, L.; Pattni, A.; Ready, D.; Wanyonyi, K.L.; White, S.; Gallagher, J.E. Evidence summary: the relationship between oral and cardiovascular disease. *Br. Dent. J.* **2017**, *222*, 381–385. [CrossRef] [PubMed]
4. Kholy, K.E.; Genco, R.J.; Van Dyke, T.E. Oral infections and cardiovascular disease. *Trends Endocrinol. Metab.* **2015**, *26*, 315–321. [CrossRef] [PubMed]
5. Preshaw, P.M.; Alba, A.L.; Herrera, D.; Jepsen, S.; Konstantinidis, A.; Makrilakis, K.; Taylor, R. Periodontitis and diabetes: a two-way relationship. *Diabetologia* **2012**, *55*, 21–31. [CrossRef] [PubMed]
6. Institute of Medicine. Advancing Oral Health in America. Available online: https://www.hrsa.gov/sites/default/files/publichealth/clinical/oralhealth/advancingoralhealth.pdf (accessed on 1 August 2019).
7. Institute of Medicine. Improving Access to Oral Health Care for Vulnerable and Underserved Populations. Available online: https://www.hrsa.gov/sites/default/files/publichealth/clinical/oralhealth/improvingaccess.pdf (accessed on 16 March 2019).
8. Choi, S.E.; Sima, C.; Pandya, A. Impact of Treating Oral Disease on Preventing Vascular Diseases: A Model-Based Cost-effectiveness Analysis of Periodontal Treatment Among Patients With Type 2 Diabetes. *Diabetes Care* **2019**. [CrossRef] [PubMed]
9. American Dental Association. Dental Care in Accountable Care Organizations: Insights from 5 Case Studies. Available online: http://www.ada.org/~{}/media/ADA/Science%20and%20Research/HPI/Files/HPIBrief_0615_1.ashx (accessed on 29 March 2019).
10. American Dental Association. Dental Care Within Accountable Care Organizations: Challenges and Opportunities. Available online: http://www.ada.org/~{}/media/ADA/Science%20and%20Research/HPI/Files/HPIBrief_0316_2.pdf (accessed on 29 March 2019).
11. Jones, J.A.; Snyder, J.J.; Gesko, D.S.; Helgeson, M.J. Integrated Medical-Dental Delivery Systems: Models in a Changing Environment and Their Implications for Dental Education. *J. Dent. Educ.* **2017**, *81*, eS21–eS29. [CrossRef] [PubMed]
12. Centers for Medicare & Medicaid Services. EHR Incentive Programs in 2015 through 2017 Health Information Exchange. Available online: https://nam.edu/integration-of-oral-health-and-primary-care-communication-coordination-and-referral/ (accessed on 25 March 2019).
13. Farhad, S.Z.; Amini, S.; Khalilian, A.; Barekatain, M.; Mafi, M.; Barekatain, M.; Rafei, E. The effect of chronic periodontitis on serum levels of tumor necrosis factor-alpha in Alzheimer disease. *Dent. Res. J.* **2014**, *11*, 549–552.
14. McKernan, S.C.; Kuthy, R.A.; Reynolds, J.C.; Tuggle, L.; Garcia, D.T. Medical-Dental Integration in Public Health Settings: An Environmental Scan. Available online: http://ppc.uiowa.edu/sites/default/files/ced_environmental_scan.pdf (accessed on 21 October 2019).
15. Crall, J.J.; Pourat, N.; Inkelas, M.; Lampron, C.; Scoville, R. Improving The Oral Health Care Capacity Of Federally Qualified Health Centers. *Health Aff.* **2016**, *35*, 2216–2223. [CrossRef] [PubMed]
16. Colorado Medical-Dental Integration Project. One Year Highlights: Colorado Medical-Dental Integration Project. Available online: https://www.deltadentalcofoundation.org/wp-content/uploads/COMDI_Handout_web.pdf (accessed on 20 March 2019).
17. Crall, J.J.; Illum, J.; Martinez, A.; Pourat, N. An Innovative Project Breaks Down Barriers to Oral Health Care for Vulnerable Young Children in Los Angeles County. *UCLA Health Policy Res* **2016**, PB2016-5. 1–8.
18. Basu, S.; Landon, B.E.; Williams, J.W., Jr.; Bitton, A.; Song, Z.; Phillips, R.S. Behavioral Health Integration into Primary Care: A Microsimulation of Financial Implications for Practices. *J. Gen. Intern. Med.* **2017**, *32*, 1330–1341. [CrossRef] [PubMed]

19. Briggs, A.H.; Weinstein, M.C.; Fenwick, E.A.; Karnon, J.; Sculpher, M.J.; Paltiel, A.D. Model parameter estimation and uncertainty analysis: A report of the ISPOR-SMDM Modeling Good Research Practices Task Force Working Group-6. *Med. Decis. Mak.* **2012**, *32*, 722–732. [CrossRef] [PubMed]
20. Robert, C.P.; Casella, G. *Introducing Monte Carlo Methods with R*; Springer Verlag: New York, NY, USA, 2009.
21. American Dental Association. Characteristics of Private Dental Practices: Selected 2017 Results from the Survey of Dental Practice. Available online: https://www.ada.org/en/science-research/health-policy-institute/data-center/dental-practice (accessed on 20 March 2019).
22. Agency for Healthcare Research and Quality. Medical Expenditure Panel Survey. Available online: https://www.meps.ahrq.gov/mepsweb/ (accessed on 20 March 2019).
23. Bureau of Labor Statistics. Occupational Outlook Handbook. Available online: https://www.bls.gov/ooh/ (accessed on 22 March 2019).
24. Medical Group Management Association. DataDive. Available online: https://www.mgma.com/data (accessed on 23 March 2019).
25. American Dental Association. Survey of Dental Practice (Annual Expenses of Operating a Private Practice). Available online: https://success.ada.org/en/practice-management/survey-of-dental-practice (accessed on 22 March 2019).
26. Delta Dental. Improving Oral Health by Integrating Medical and Dental Care—EMR/EDR. Available online: http://medicaldentalintegration.org/building-mdi-models/building-co-mdi-space/ehredr/ (accessed on 5 December 2019).
27. American Dental Association. The Real Cost of Owning a Dental Practice. Available online: http://marketplace.ada.org/blog/the-real-cost-of-owning-a-dental-practice/ (accessed on 20 March 2019).
28. Liu, C.F.; Rubenstein, L.V.; Kirchner, J.E.; Fortney, J.C.; Perkins, M.W.; Ober, S.K.; Pyne, J.M.; Chaney, E.F. Organizational cost of quality improvement for depression care. *Health Serv. Res.* **2009**, *44*, 225–244. [CrossRef] [PubMed]
29. Silk, H.; Sachs Leicher, E.; Alvarado, V.; Cote, E.; Cote, S. A multi-state initiative to implement pediatric oral health in primary care practice and clinical education. *J. Public Health Dent.* **2018**, *78*, 25–31. [CrossRef] [PubMed]
30. The Physicians Foundation. Survey of America's Physician. Available online: https://physiciansfoundation.org/wp-content/uploads/2018/09/physicians-survey-results-final-2018.pdf (accessed on 24 April 2019).
31. American Dental Association. Code on Dental Procedures and Nomenclature (CDT Code). Available online: https://www.ada.org/en/publications/cdt (accessed on 20 March 2019).
32. Maryland Department of Health. Maryland Medicaid Dental Fee Schedule and Procedure Codes. Available online: https://mmcp.health.maryland.gov/Documents/2018%20CDT%20Fee%20Schedule%20FINAL%20 (accessed on 14 December 2019).
33. American Dental Association. Income, Gross Billings, and Expenses: Selected 2017 Results from the Survey of Dental Practice. Available online: https://www.ada.org/en/science-research/health-policy-institute/dental-statistics/income-billing-and-other-dentistry-statistics (accessed on 20 March 2019).
34. American Dental Association. Employment of Dental Practice Personnel: Selected 2013 Results from the Survey of Dental Practice. Available online: https://www.ada.org/en/science-research/health-policy-institute/data-center/dental-practice (accessed on 2 April 2019).
35. Florida Blue Dental. Oral Health for Overall Health. Available online: https://www.floridabluedental.com/members/oral-health-for-overall-health/ (accessed on 12 February 2019).
36. United Concordia Dental. Smile for Health—Wellness. Available online: https://www.unitedconcordia.com/dental-insurance/employer/dental-plans/innovative-solutions-dental-plans/product-smile-for-health-wellness/ (accessed on 12 February 2019).
37. Delta Dental. SmileWay Wellness Benefits. Available online: https://www.deltadentalins.com/individuals/guidance/smileway-wellness-benefits.html (accessed on 12 February 2019).
38. American Dental Association. Supply and Profile of Dentists. Available online: https://www.ada.org/en/science-research/health-policy-institute/data-center/supply-and-profile-of-dentists (accessed on 30 March 2019).
39. National Association of Community Health Centers. Community Health Center Chartbook. Available online: http://www.nachc.org/wp-content/uploads/2017/06/Chartbook2017.pdf (accessed on 20 April 2019).

40. Gillis. K.D. *Physicians' Patient Mix—A Snapshot from the 2016 Benchmark Survey and Changes Associated with the ACA*. Available online: https://www.ama-assn.org/sites/ama-assn.org/files/corp/media-browser/public/health-policy/PRP-2017-physician-benchmark-survey-patient-mix.pdf (accessed on 22 March 2020).
41. Kalenderian, E.; Halamka, J.D.; Spallek, H. An EHR with Teeth. *Appl. Clin. Inform.* **2016**, *7*, 425–429. [CrossRef] [PubMed]
42. Tan, K.B.; Earn Lee, C. Integration of Primary Care with Hospital Services for Sustainable Universal Health Coverage in Singapore. *Health Syst. Reform* **2019**, *5*, 18–23. [CrossRef] [PubMed]
43. Martinez-Alvarez, C.; Sanz, M.; Berthold, P. Basic sciences education in the dental curriculum in Southern Europe. *Eur. J. Dent. Educ.* **2001**, *5*, 63–66. [CrossRef] [PubMed]
44. Nasseh, K.; Vujicic, M.; Glick, M. The Relationship between Periodontal Interventions and Healthcare Costs and Utilization. Evidence from an Integrated Dental, Medical, and Pharmacy Commercial Claims Database. *Health Econ.* **2017**, *26*, 519–527. [CrossRef] [PubMed]
45. Jeffcoat, M.K.; Jeffcoat, R.L.; Gladowski, P.A.; Bramson, J.B.; Blum, J.J. Impact of periodontal therapy on general health: Evidence from insurance data for five systemic conditions. *Am. J. Prev. Med.* **2014**, *47*, 166–174. [CrossRef] [PubMed]
46. Centers for Medicare & Medicaid Services. Medicaid Analytic eXtract (MAX) Chartbooks. Available online: https://www.cms.gov/Research-Statistics-Data-and-Systems/Computer-Data-and-Systems/MedicaidDataSourcesGenInfo/MAX_Chartbooks.html (accessed on 29 March 2019).

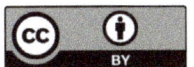

© 2020 by the authors. Licensee MDPI, Basel, Switzerland. This article is an open access article distributed under the terms and conditions of the Creative Commons Attribution (CC BY) license (http://creativecommons.org/licenses/by/4.0/).

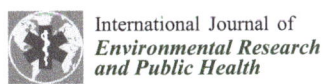

Review

Current Applications, Opportunities, and Limitations of AI for 3D Imaging in Dental Research and Practice

Kuofeng Hung [1], Andy Wai Kan Yeung [1], Ray Tanaka [1] and Michael M. Bornstein [1,2,*]

[1] Oral and Maxillofacial Radiology, Applied Oral Sciences and Community Dental Care, Faculty of Dentistry, The University of Hong Kong, Hong Kong 999077, China; hungkf@connect.hku.hk (K.H.); ndyeung@hku.hk (A.W.K.Y.); rayt3@hku.hk (R.T.)
[2] Department of Oral Health & Medicine, University Center for Dental Medicine Basel UZB, University of Basel, 4058 Basel, Switzerland
* Correspondence: michael.bornstein@unibas.ch; Tel.: +41-(0)61-267-25-45

Received: 19 March 2020; Accepted: 16 June 2020; Published: 19 June 2020

Abstract: The increasing use of three-dimensional (3D) imaging techniques in dental medicine has boosted the development and use of artificial intelligence (AI) systems for various clinical problems. Cone beam computed tomography (CBCT) and intraoral/facial scans are potential sources of image data to develop 3D image-based AI systems for automated diagnosis, treatment planning, and prediction of treatment outcome. This review focuses on current developments and performance of AI for 3D imaging in dentomaxillofacial radiology (DMFR) as well as intraoral and facial scanning. In DMFR, machine learning-based algorithms proposed in the literature focus on three main applications, including automated diagnosis of dental and maxillofacial diseases, localization of anatomical landmarks for orthodontic and orthognathic treatment planning, and general improvement of image quality. Automatic recognition of teeth and diagnosis of facial deformations using AI systems based on intraoral and facial scanning will very likely be a field of increased interest in the future. The review is aimed at providing dental practitioners and interested colleagues in healthcare with a comprehensive understanding of the current trend of AI developments in the field of 3D imaging in dental medicine.

Keywords: artificial intelligence; AI; machine learning; ML; cone beam computed tomography (CBCT); intraoral scanning; facial scanning

1. Introduction

Artificial intelligence (AI) is generally defined as intelligent computer programs capable of learning and applying knowledge to accomplish complex tasks such as to predict treatment outcomes, recognize objects, and answer questions [1]. Nowadays, AI technologies are widespread and penetrate many applications of our daily life, such as Amazon's online shopping recommendations, Facebook's image recognition, Netflix's streaming videos, and the smartphone's voice assistant [2]. For such daily life applications, it is characteristic that the initial use of an AI-driven system will give a more generalized outcome based on big data, and after repeated use by the individual, it will gradually present a more adapted and personalized outcome in accordance with the user's characteristics. The remarkable success of AI in various fields of our daily life has inspired and is stimulating the development of AI systems in the field of medicine and, also, more specifically, dental medicine [3,4].

Radiology is deemed to be the front door for AI into medicine as digitally coded diagnostic images are more easily translated into computer language [5]. Thus, diagnostic images are seen as one of the primary sources of data used to develop AI systems for the purpose of an automated prediction of disease risk (such as osteoporotic bone fractures [6]), detection of pathologies (such as coronary artery calcification as a predictor for atherosclerosis [7]), and diagnosis of disease (such as skin cancers in dermatology [8]). Machine learning is a key component of AI, and commonly applied to develop image-based AI systems. Through a synergism between radiologists and the medical AI system used, increased work efficiency and more precise outcomes regarding the final diagnosis of various diseases are expected to be achieved [9,10].

In the field of dental and maxillofacial radiology (DMFR), reports on AI models used for diagnostic purposes and treatment planning cover a wide range of clinical applications, including automated localization of craniofacial anatomical structures/pathological changes, classification of maxillofacial cysts and/or tumors, and diagnosis of caries and periodontal lesions [11]. According to the literature related to clinical applications of AI in DMFR, most of the proposed machine learning algorithms were developed using two-dimensional (2D) diagnostic images, such as periapical, panoramic, and cephalometric radiographs [11]. However, 2D images have several limitations, including image magnification and distortion, superimposition of anatomical structures, and the lack of three-dimensional information for relevant landmarks/pathological changes. These may lower the diagnostic accuracy of the AI models trained using only 2D images [12]. For example, a 2D image-based AI model built for the detection of periodontal bone defects might not be able to detect three-walled bony defects, loss of buccal/oral cortical bone plates, or bone defects around overlapping teeth. Three-dimensional (3D) imaging techniques, including cone beam computed tomography (CBCT), as well as intraoral and facial scanning systems, are increasingly used in dental practice. CBCT imaging allows for the visualization and assessment of bony anatomic structures and/or pathological changes in 3D with high diagnostic accuracy and precision. The use of CBCT is of great help when conventional 2D imaging techniques do not provide sufficient information for diagnosis and treatment planning purposes [13]. Intraoral and facial scanning systems are reported to be reproducible and reliable to capture 3D soft-tissue images that can be used for digital treatment planning systems [14,15]. CBCT and intraoral/facial scans are considered as an ideal data source for developing AI models to overcome the limitations of 2D image-based algorithms [12,15]. Thus, the aim of this review is to describe current developments and to assess the performance of AI models for 3D imaging in DMFR, as well as intraoral and facial scanning.

2. Current Use of AI for 3D Imaging in DMFR

A literature search was conducted using PubMed to identify all existing studies of AI applications for 3D imaging in DMFR and intraoral/facial scanning. The search was conducted without restriction on the publication period but was limited to studies in English. The keywords used for the search were combinations of terms including "artificial intelligence", "AI", "machine learning", "deep learning", "convolutional neural networks", "automatic", "automated", "three-dimensional imaging", "3D imaging", "cone beam computed tomography", "CBCT", "three-dimensional scan", "3D scan", "intraoral scan", "intraoral scanning", "facial scan", "facial scanning", and/or "dentistry". Reviews, conference papers, and studies using clinical/nonclinical image data were eligible for the initial screening process. Initially, titles of the identified studies were manually screened, and subsequently, abstracts of the relevant studies were read to identify studies for further full-text reading. Furthermore, references of included articles were examined to identify further relevant articles. As a result, approximately 650 publications were initially screened, and 23 publications were eventually included in the present review for data extraction (details provided in Tables 1 and 2).

The methodological quality of the included studies was evaluated using the assessment criteria proposed by Hung et al. [11]. For proposed AI models for diagnosis/classification of a certain condition, four studies [16–19] were rated as having a "high" or an "unclear" risk of concern in the domain of subject selection because the testing dataset only consisted of images from subjects with the condition of interest. With regard to the selection of reference standards, all studies were considered as "low" risk of concern as expert judgment and clinical or pathological examination was applied as the reference standard. Concerns regarding the risk of bias were relatively high in the domain of index test, as ten [16,17,20–27] of the included studies did not test their AI models on independent images unused for developing the algorithms.

Table 1 exhibits the included studies regarding the use of AI for 3D imaging in DMFR. These studies focused on three main applications, including automated diagnosis of dental and maxillofacial diseases [16–20,28–32], localization of anatomical landmarks for orthodontic and orthognathic treatment planning [21,22,33–35], and improvement of image quality [23,36].

2.1. Automated Diagnosis of Dental and Maxillofacial Diseases

The basic principle of the learning algorithms for diagnostic purposes is to explore associations between the input image and output diagnosis. Theoretically, a machine learning algorithm is initially built using hand-crafted detectors of image features in a predefined framework, subsequently trained with the training data, iteratively adapted to minimize the error at the output, and eventually tested with the unseen testing data to verify its validity [37]. Deep learning, a subset of machine learning, is able to automatically learn to extract relevant image features without the requirement of the manual design of image feature detectors, which is currently considered as the most suitable method to develop image-based diagnostic AI models [12].

The workflow of the proposed machine learning algorithms for diagnostic purpose can be mainly categorized as (see Figure 1).

1. Input image data;
2. Image preprocessing;
3. Selection of the region of interest (ROI);
4. Segmentation of lesions;
5. Extraction of selected texture features in the segmented lesions;
6. Analysis of the extracted features;
7. Output of the diagnosis or classification.

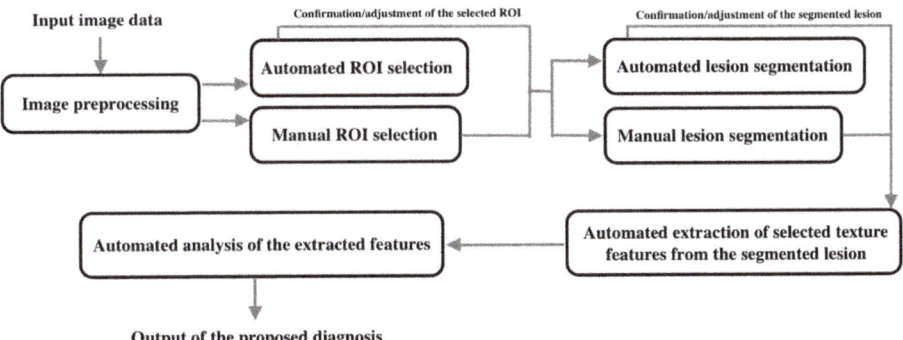

Figure 1. The workflow of the proposed machine learning algorithms for diagnostic purposes.

Table 1. Characteristics of studies describing machine learning-based artificial intelligence (AI) models applied in dentomaxillofacial radiology (DMFR).

Author (Year)	Application	Imaging Modality	AI Technique	Image Data Set Used to Develop the AI Model	Independent Testing Image Data Set / Validation Technique	Performance
\multicolumn{7}{c}{Diagnosis of Dental and Maxillofacial Diseases}					
Okada [16] (2015)	Diagnosis of periapical cysts and granuloma	CBCT	LDA	28 scans from patients with periapical cysts or granuloma	7-fold CV	94.1% (accuracy)
Abdolali [17] (2017)	Diagnosis of radicular cysts, dentigerous cysts, and keratocysts	CBCT	SVM; SDA	96 scans from patients with radicular cysts, dentigerous cysts, or keratocysts	3-fold CV	94.29–96.48% (accuracy)
Yilmaz [18] (2017)	Diagnosis of periapical cysts and keratocysts	CBCT	k-NN; Naïve Bayes; Decision tree; Random forest; NN; SVM	50 scans from patients with cysts or tumors	10-fold CV/LOOCV	94–100% (accuracy)
				25 scans from patients with cysts or tumors	25 scans from patients with cysts or tumors	
Lee [19] (2020)	Diagnosis of periapical cysts, dentigerous cysts, and keratocysts	Panoramic radiography and CBCT	CNN	912 panoramic images and 789 CBCT scans	228 panoramic images and 197 CBCT scans	Panoramic radiography 0.847 (AUC); 88.2% (sensitivity); 77.0% (specificity) CBCT 0.914 (AUC); 96.1% (sensitivity); 77.1% (specificity)
Orhan [28] (2020)	Diagnosis of periapical pathology	CBCT	CNN	3900 scans acquired using multiple FOVs from 2800 patients with periapical lesions and 1100 subjects without periapical lesions	109 scans acquired using multiple FOVs from 153 patients with periapical lesions	92.8% (accuracy)
Abdolali [29] (2019)	Diagnosis of radiolucent lesion, maxillary sinus perforation, unerupted tooth, and root fracture	CBCT	Symmetry-based analysis model	686 scans acquired using a large FOV (12 × 15 × 15 cm^3), collected from several dental imaging centers in Iran	459 scans acquired using a large FOV (12 × 15 × 15 cm^3), collected from several dental imaging centers in Iran	0.85–0.92 (DSC)

Table 1. Cont.

Author (Year)	Application	Imaging Modality	AI Technique	Image Data Set Used to Develop the AI Model	Independent Testing Image Data Set / Validation Technique	Performance
Johari [30] (2017)	Detection of vertical root fractures	Periapical radiography and CBCT	CNN	180 periapical radiographs and 180 CBCT scans of the extracted teeth	60 periapical radiographs and 60 CBCT scans of the extracted teeth	Periapical radiography 70.0% (accuracy); 97.8% (sensitivity); 67.6% (specificity) CBCT 96.6% (accuracy); 93.3% (sensitivity); 100% (specificity)
Kise [32] (2019)	Diagnosis of Sjögren's syndrome	CT	CNN	400 scans (200 from 20 SjS patients and 200 from 20 control subjects) acquired using a large FOV	100 scans (50 from 5 SjS patients and 50 from 5 control subjects) acquired using a large FOV	96.0% (accuracy); 100% (sensitivity); 92.0% (specificity)
Kann [31] (2018)	Detection of lymph node metastasis and extranodal extension in patients with head and neck cancer	Contrast-enhanced CT	CNN	Images of 2875 CT-segmented lymph node samples with correlating pathology labels	Images of 131 lymph nodes (76 negative and 55 positive)	0.91 (AUC)
Ariji [20] (2019)	Detection of lymph node metastasis in patients with oral cancer	Contrast-enhanced CT	CNN	Images of 441 lymph nodes (314 negative and 127 positive) from 45 patients	5-fold CV	78.2% (accuracy); 75.4% (sensitivity); 81.0% (specificity), 0.80 (AUC)
Localization of Anatomical Landmarks for Orthodontic and Orthognathic Treatment Planning							
Cheng [33] (2011)	Localization of the odontoid process of the second vertebra	CBCT	Random forest	50 scans	23 scans	3.15 mm (mean deviation)
Shahidi [34] (2014)	Localization of 14 anatomical landmarks	CBCT	Feature-based and voxel similarity-based algorithms	8 scans acquired using a large FOV from subjects aged 10–45 years	20 scans acquired using a large FOV from subjects aged 10–45 years	3.40 mm (mean deviation)

Table 1. Cont.

Author (Year)	Application	Imaging Modality	AI Technique	Image Data Set Used to Develop the AI Model	Independent Testing Image Data Set / Validation Technique	Performance
Montufar [21] (2018)	Localization of 18 anatomical landmarks	CBCT	Active shape model	24 scans acquired using a large FOV	LOOCV	3.64 mm (mean deviation)
Montufar [22] (2018)	Localization of 18 anatomical landmarks	CBCT	Active shape model	24 scans acquired using a large FOV	LOOCV	2.51 mm (mean deviation)
Torosdagli [35] (2019)	Localization of 9 anatomical landmarks	CBCT	CNN	50 scans	48 scans	0.9382 (DSC); 93.42% (sensitivity); 99.97% (specificity),
Improvement of Image Quality							
Park [36] (2018)	Improvement of image resolution	CT	CNN	52 scans	13 scans	The CNN network can yield high-resolution images based on low-resolution images
Minnema [23] (2019)	Segmentation of CBCT scans affected by metal artifacts	CBCT	CNN	20 scans	Leave-2-out CV	The CNN network can accurately segment bony structures in CBCT scans affected by metal artifacts
Other							
Miki [38] (2017)	Tooth classification	CBCT	CNN	42 scans with the diameter of the FOV ranged from 5.1 to 20 cm	10 scans with the diameter of the FOV ranged from 5.1 to 20 cm	88.8% (accuracy)

AI, artificial intelligence; AUC, area under the receiver operating characteristic curve; CBCT, cone beam computed tomography; CNN, convolutional neural network; CT, computed tomography; CV, cross validation; DSC, dice similarity coefficient; FOV, field of view; k-NN, k-nearest neighbors; LDA, linear discriminant analysis; LOOCV, leave-one-out cross-validation; NN, neural network; SDA, sparse discriminant analysis; SjS, Sjögren's syndrome; SVM, support vector machine.

Some of the proposed machine learning algorithms were not fully automated and required manual operation/adjustment for the ROI selection or lesion segmentation. Okada et al. proposed a semiautomatic machine learning algorithm, using CBCT images to classify periapical cysts and granulomas [16]. This algorithm requires users to segment the target lesion before it proceeds to the next step (feature extraction). Yilmaz et al. proposed a semiautomatic algorithm, using CBCT images to classify periapical cysts and keratocysts [18]. In this algorithm, detection and segmentation of lesions are required to be performed manually. The users need to mark the lesion on different cross-sectional planes to predefine the volume of interest containing the lesion. Manual segmentation of cystic lesions on multiple CBCT slices is time-consuming, which limits the efficiency of the algorithms and also their implementation for routine clinical use. Lee et al. proposed deep learning algorithms, respectively, using panoramic radiographs and CBCT images for the detection and diagnosis of periapical cysts, dentigerous cysts, and keratocysts [19]. It was reported that automatic edge detection techniques can segment cystic lesions more efficiently and accurately than manual segmentation. This can shorten the execution time for the segmentation step and improve the usability of the proposed algorithms for clinical practice. Moreover, higher diagnostic accuracy was reported for CBCT image-based algorithms in comparison with panoramic image-based ones. This may result from a higher accuracy in detecting the lesion boundary in 3D and more quantitative features extracted from the voxel units. Abdolali et al. proposed an algorithm based on asymmetry analysis using CBCT images to automatically segment cystic lesions, including dentigerous cysts, radicular cysts, and keratocysts [39]. The algorithm exhibited promising performance with high true-positives and low false-positives. However, its limitations include a relatively low detection rate for small cysts, imperfect segmentation of keratocysts without well-defined boundaries, and the incapability of dealing with symmetric cysts crossing the midsagittal plane. Based on the proposed segmentation algorithm, Abdolali et al. developed another AI model using CBCT images to automatically classify dentigerous cysts, radicular cysts, and keratocysts [17]. This model exhibited high classification accuracies ranging from 94.29% to 96.48%. Subsequently, Abdolali et al. further proposed a fully automated medical-content-based image retrieval system for the diagnosis of four maxillofacial lesions/conditions, including radiolucent lesions, maxillary sinus perforation, unerupted teeth, and root fractures [29]. In this novel system, an improved version of a previously proposed segmentation algorithm [39] was incorporated. The diagnostic accuracy of the proposed system was 90%, with a significantly reduced segmentation time of three minutes per case. It was stated that this system is more effective than previous models proposed in the literature, and is promising for introduction into clinical practice in the near future.

Orhan et al. verified the performance of a deep learning algorithm using CBCT images to detect and volumetrically measure periapical lesions [28]. A detection rate of 92.8% and a significant positive correlation between the automated and manual measurements were reported. The differences between manual and automated measurements are mainly due to inaccurate lesion segmentation. Because of low soft-tissue contrast in CBCT images, the deep learning algorithm exhibits difficulties in perfectly distinguishing the lesion area from neighboring soft tissue when buccal/oral cortical perforations or endo-perio lesions occur. Johari et al. proposed deep learning algorithms using periapical and CBCT images to detect vertical root fractures [30]. The results showed that the proposed model resulted in higher diagnostic performance for CBCT images than periapicals. Furthermore, some studies have reported on the application of deep learning algorithms for the diagnosis of Sjögren's syndrome or lymph node metastasis. Kise et al. proposed a deep learning algorithm using CT images to assist inexperienced radiologists to semiautomatically diagnose Sjögren's syndrome [32]. The results exhibited that the diagnostic performance of the deep learning algorithm is comparable to experienced radiologists and is significantly higher than for inexperienced radiologists. The main limitation of the proposed algorithm is its semiautomatic nature, requiring manual image segmentation prior to performing automated diagnosis. For further ease and implementation in daily routine, a completely automated segmentation of the region of the parotid gland should be developed and incorporated into a fully automated diagnostic system. Kann et al. and Ariji et al., respectively, proposed deep learning algorithms using contrast-enhanced CT images to semiautomatically identify nodal metastasis in patients with oral/head and neck cancer [20,31]. The user of the respective programs is required to manually segment the contour of lymph nodes on multiple CT slices. Excellent performance was reported for both algorithms proposed, which was close to or even surpassed the diagnostic accuracy of experienced radiologists. Therefore, these deep learning algorithms have the potential to help guide oral/head and neck cancer patient management. Future investigations should focus on the development of a fully automated identification system to avoid manual segmentation of lymph nodes. This can significantly improve the efficiency of the AI system used and could enable wider use of this system in community clinics.

2.2. Automated Localization of Anatomical Landmarks for Orthodontic and Orthognathic Treatment Planning

The correct analysis of craniofacial anatomy and facial proportions is the basis of successful orthodontic and orthognathic treatment. Traditional orthodontic analysis is generally conducted on 2D cephalometric radiographs, which can be less accurate due to image magnification, superimposition of structures, inappropriate X-ray projection angle, and patient position. Since CBCT was introduced in dental medicine, 3D diagnosis and virtual treatment planning have been assessed as a more accurate option for orthodontic and orthognathic treatment [40]. Although 3D orthodontic analysis can be performed by a computer-aided digital tracing approach, it still requires orthodontists to manually locate anatomical landmarks on multiple CBCT slices. The manual localization process is tedious and time-consuming, which may currently discourage orthodontists from switching to a fully digital workflow. Cheng et al. proposed the first machine learning algorithm to automatically localize one key landmark on CBCT images and reported promising results [33]. Subsequently, a series of machine learning algorithms were developed for automated localization of several anatomical landmarks and analysis of dentofacial deformity. Shahidi et al. proposed a machine-learning algorithm to automatically locate 14 craniofacial landmarks on CBCT images, whereas the mean deviation (3.40 mm) for all of the automatically identified landmarks was higher than the mean deviation (1.41 mm) for the manually detected ones [34]. Montufar et al. proposed two different automatic landmark localization systems, respectively, based on active shape models and a hybrid approach using active shape models followed by a 3D knowledge-based searching algorithm [21,22]. The mean deviation (2.51 mm) for all of the automatically identified landmarks in the hybrid system was lower than that of the system only using active shape models (3.64 mm). Despite less localization deviation, the performance of automated localization in the proposed systems is still not accurate enough to meet clinical requirements. Therefore, the existing AI systems can only be recommended for the use of preliminary localization of the orthodontic landmarks, but manual correction is still necessary prior to further orthodontic analyses. This may be the main limitation of these AI systems and this needs to be improved for future clinical dissemination and use.

Orthodontic and orthognathic treatments in patients with craniofacial deformities are challenging. The aforementioned AI systems may not be able to effectively deal with such patients. Torosdagli et al. proposed a novel deep learning algorithm applied for fully automated mandible segmentation and landmarking in craniofacial anomalies on CBCT images [35]. The proposed algorithm allows for orthodontic analysis in patients with craniofacial deformities and showed excellent performance with a sensitivity of 93.42% and specificity of 99.97%. Future studies should consider widening the field of applications for AI systems, especially for different patient populations.

2.3. Automated Improvement of Image Quality

Radiation dose protection is of paramount importance in medicine and also for DMFR. It is reported that medical radiation exposure is the largest artificial radiation source and represents approximately 14% of the total annual dose of ionizing radiation for individuals [41]. Computed tomography (CT) imaging is widely used to assist clinical diagnosis in various fields of medicine. Reducing the scanning slice thickness is the general option to enhance the resolution of CT images. However, this will increase the noise level as well as radiation dose exposure to the patient. High-resolution CT images are recommended only when low-resolution CT images do not provide sufficient information for diagnosis and treatment planning purposes in individual cases [42]. The balance between the radiation dose and CT image resolution is the biggest concern for radiologists. To address this issue, Park et al. proposed a deep learning algorithm to enhance the thick-slice CT image resolution similar to that of a thin slice [36]. It is reported that the noise level of the enhanced CT images is even lower than the original images. Therefore, this algorithm has the potential to be a useful tool for enhancing the image resolution for CT scans as well as reducing the radiation dose and noise level. It is expected that such an algorithm can further be developed for CBCT scans.

The presence of metal artifacts in CT/CBCT images is another critical issue that can obscure neighboring anatomical structures and interfere with disease diagnosis. In dental medicine, metal artifacts are not uncommon in CBCT images due to materials used for dental restorations or orthodontic purposes. These metal artifacts not only interfere with disease diagnosis but, in some cases, impede the image segmentation of the teeth and bony structures in the maxilla and mandible for computer-guided treatment. Minnema et al. proposed a deep learning algorithm based on a mixed-scale dense convolutional neural network for the segmentation of teeth and bone on CBCT images affected by metal artifacts [23]. It is reported that the proposed algorithm can accurately classify metal artifacts as background and segment teeth and bony structures. The promising results prove that a convolutional neural network is capable of extracting the characteristic features in CBCT voxel units that cannot be distinguished by human eyes.

2.4. Other Applications

In addition to the above AI applications, automated tooth detection, classification, and numbering are also fields of great interest, and they have the potential to simplify the process of filling out digital dental charts [43]. Miki et al. developed a deep learning algorithm based on a convolutional neural network to automatically classify tooth types based on CBCT images [38]. Although this algorithm was designed for automated filling of dental charts for forensic identification purposes, it may also be valuable to incorporate it into the digital treatment planning system, especially for use in implantology and prosthetics. For example, such an application may contribute to the automated identification of missing teeth for the diagnosis and planning of implants or other prosthetic treatments.

3. Current Use of AI for Intraoral 3D Imaging and Facial Scanning

In recent years, computer-aided design and manufacturing (CAD/CAM) technology have been widely used in various fields of dentistry, especially in implantology, prosthetics, orthodontics, and maxillofacial surgery. For example, CAD/CAM technology can be used for the fabrication of surgical implant guides, provisional/definitive restorations, orthodontic appliances, and maxillofacial surgical templates. Most of these applications are based on 3D hard and soft tissue images generated by CBCT and optical scanning (such as intraoral/facial scanning and scanning of dental casts/impressions). Intraoral scanning is the most accurate method of digitalizing the 3D contour of teeth and gingiva [44]. As a result, the intraoral scanning technique is now gradually replacing the scanning of dental casts or impressions and is also frequently used in CAD/CAM systems. Tooth segmentation is a critical step, which is usually performed manually by trained dental practitioners in a digital workflow to design and fabricate restorations and orthodontic appliances. However, manual segmentation is time-consuming, poorly reproducible, and limited due to human error, which may eventually have a negative influence on treatment outcome. Ghazvinian Zanjani et al. and Kim et al., respectively, developed deep learning algorithms for automated tooth segmentation on digitalized 3D dental surface models resulting in high segmentation precision (Table 2) [24,45]. These algorithms can speed up the digital workflow and reduce human error. Furthermore, Lian et al. proposed an automated tooth labeling algorithm based on intraoral scanning [25]. This algorithm can simplify the process of tooth position rearrangements in orthodontic treatment planning.

Table 2. Characteristics of the machine learning-based AI models based on intraoral and facial scanning.

Author (Year)	Application	Imaging Modality	AI Technique	Image Data Set Used to Develop the AI Model	Independent Testing Image Data Set/Validation Technique	Performance
Ghazvinian Zanjani [24] (2019)	Tooth segmentation	Intraoral scanning	CNN	120 scans, comprising 60 upper jaws and 60 lower jaws.	5-fold CV	0.94 (intersection over union score)
Kim [45] (2020)	Tooth segmentation	Intraoral scanning	Generative adversarial network	10,000 cropped images	Approximate 350 cropped images	An average improvement of 0.004 mm in the tooth segmentation
Lian [25] (2020)	Tooth labelling	Intraoral scanning	CNN	30 scans of upper jaws	5-fold CV	0.894 to 0.970 (DSC)
Liu [27] (2016)	Identification of Autism Spectrum Disorder	Facial scanning	SVM	87 scans from children with and without Autism Spectrum Disorder	LOOCV	88.51% (accuracy)
Knoops [26] (2019)	Diagnosis and planning in plastic and reconstructive surgery	Facial scanning	Machine-learning-based 3D morphable model	4261 scans from healthy subjects and orthognathic patients	LOOCV	Diagnosis 95.5% (sensitivity); 95.2% (specificity) Surgical simulation 1.1 ± 0.3 mm (accuracy)

3D, three-dimensional; AI, artificial intelligence; CV, cross-validation; DSC, dice similarity coefficient; LOOCV, leave-one-out cross-validation; SVM, support vector machine.

Currently, only a few studies have reported on the use of machine learning techniques based on facial scanning (Table 2). Knoops et al. proposed an AI 3D-morphable model based on facial scanning to automatically analyze facial shape features for diagnosis and planning in plastic and reconstructive surgery [26]. In addition, this model is also able to predict patient-specific postoperative outcomes. The proposed model may improve the efficiency and accuracy in diagnosis and treatment planning, and help preoperative communication with the patient. However, this model can only perform an analysis based on 3D facial scanning alone. As facial scanning is unable to acquire volumetric bone data, the information about the underlying skeletal structures cannot be analyzed by this model. An updated model that can perform the analysis simultaneously on facial soft tissue and skeletal structures will be more realistic and probably more effective for clinical use.

Interestingly, facial scanning techniques in combination with AI can also be used for the diagnosis of neurodevelopmental disorders, such as autism spectrum disorder (ASD). Liu et al. explored the possibility of using a machine learning algorithm based on facial scanning to identify ASD and showed promising results with an accuracy of 88.51% (Table 2) [27]. This algorithm could be a supportive tool for the screening and diagnosis of ASD in clinical practice.

4. Limitations of the Included Studies

While the AI models proposed in the included studies have shown promising performance, several limitations are worth noting, which may affect the reliability of the proposed models. First, most of the proposed AI models were developed using a small number of images collected from the same institution over one defined time period (see details in Tables 1–3). Additionally, some classification models were only trained and tested using images from subjects with confirmed diseases (Table 3). These limitations might result in a risk of overfitting and a too optimistic appraisal of the proposed models. In addition, the images used to develop the algorithms might very likely be captured using the same device and imaging protocols, resulting in a lack of data heterogeneity (Table 3). This might cause a lack of generalizability and reliability of the proposed models and can result in inferior performance in clinical practice settings due to differences in variables, including devices, imaging protocols, and patient populations [46]. Thus, these models may still need to be verified by using adequate heterogeneous data collected from different dental institutions prior to being transferred and implemented into clinical practice.

Table 3. Conclusions and limitations of the included studies.

Author (Year)	Conclusion	Limitations (Risk of Bias *)
Okada [16] (2015)	The proposed model may assist clinicians to accurately differentiate periapical lesions.	• A small training dataset *; Lacking data heterogeneity *; Dataset only consisted of scans from subjects with the condition of interest *; Lacking independent unseen testing data *; Manual ROI selection; Long execution time.
Abdolali [17] (2017)	The proposed model can improve the accuracy of the diagnosis of dentigerous cysts, radicular cysts, and keratocysts, and may have a significant impact on future AI diagnostic systems.	• A small training dataset *; Lacking data heterogeneity *; Dataset only consisted of scans from subjects with the condition of interest *; Lacking independent unseen testing data *.
Yilmaz [18] (2017)	Periapical cysts and keratocysts can be classified with high accuracy with the proposed model. It can also contribute to the field of automated diagnosis of periapical lesions.	• A small training dataset *; Lacking data heterogeneity *; Dataset only consisted of scans from subjects with the condition of interest *; Manual detection and segmentation of lesions.
Lee [19] (2020)	Periapical cysts, dentigerous cysts, and keratocysts can be effectively detected and diagnosed with the proposed deep CNN algorithm, but the diagnosis of these lesions using radiological data alone, without histological examination, is still challenging.	• A relatively small training dataset *; Dataset only consisted of scans from subjects with the condition of interest *; Manual ROI selection; Potential overfitting problem in the training procedure *.
Orhan [28] (2020)	The proposed deep learning systems can be useful for detection and volumetric measurement of periapical lesions. The diagnostic performance was comparable to that of an oral and maxillofacial radiologist.	• Relatively inaccurate segmentation of lesions in close contact with neighboring soft tissue
Abdolali [29] (2019)	The proposed system is effective and can automatically diagnose various maxillofacial lesions/conditions. It can facilitate the introduction of content-based image retrieval in clinical CBCT applications.	• Relatively inaccurate detection of symmetric lesions
Johari [30] (2017)	The proposed deep learning model can be used for the diagnosis of vertical root fractures on CBCT images of endodontically treated and also vital teeth. With the aid of the model, the use of CBCT images is more effective than periapical radiographs.	• A small training dataset *; Ex-vivo data only containing sound extracted premolars *; Lacking data heterogeneity *; Unknown diagnostic performance on multirooted teeth and teeth with caries or filling materials *.

Table 3. *Cont.*

Author (Year)	Conclusion	Limitations (Risk of Bias *)
Kise [32] (2019)	The deep learning model showed high diagnostic accuracy for SjS, which is comparable to that of experienced radiologists. It is suggested that the model could be used to assist the diagnosis of SjS, especially for inexperienced radiologists.	• A small training dataset *; Lacking data heterogeneity *; Lacking subjects with other pathological changes of the parotid gland in the control subjects *; Manual ROI segmentation.
Kann [31] (2018)	The proposed deep learning model has the potential for use as a clinical decision-making tool to help guide head and neck cancer patient management.	• The process of individual lymph node CT labeling in correlation with pathology reports is subject to some degree of uncertainty and subjectivity *; Only lymph nodes for which a definitive correlation could be made were included in the labeled dataset, potentially biasing the dataset to those nodes that could be definitively correlated with pathologic report *.
Ariji [20] (2019)	The proposed deep learning model yielded diagnostic results comparable to that of radiologists, which suggests that the model may be valuable for diagnostic support.	• A small training dataset *; Lacking data heterogeneity *; Lacking independent unseen testing data *; Manual ROI segmentation;
Cheng [33] (2011)	The proposed model can efficiently assist clinicians in locating the odontoid process of the second vertebra.	• A small training dataset *; Lacking data heterogeneity *; Inaccurate localization performance.
Shahidi [34] (2014)	The localization performance of the proposed model was acceptable with a mean deviation of 3.40 mm for all automatically identified landmarks.	• A small training dataset *; Lacking data heterogeneity *; Inaccurate localization performance.
Montufar [21] (2018)	The proposed algorithm for automatically locating landmarks on CBCT volumes seems to be useful for 3D cephalometric analysis.	• A small training dataset *; Lacking data heterogeneity *; Lacking independent unseen testing data *; Inaccurate localization performance.
Montufar [22] (2018)	The proposed hybrid algorithm for automatic landmarking on CBCT volumes seems to be potentially useful for 3D cephalometric analysis.	• A small training dataset *; Lacking data heterogeneity *; Lacking independent unseen testing data *; Relatively inaccurate localization performance.
Torosdagli [35] (2019)	The proposed deep learning algorithm allows for orthodontic analysis in patients with craniofacial deformities exhibiting excellent performance.	• A small training dataset *; Lacking data heterogeneity *; Analysis of pseudo-3D images instead of fully 3D images *;

Table 3. Cont.

Author (Year)	Conclusion	Limitations (Risk of Bias *)
Park [36] (2018)	The proposed deep learning algorithm is useful for super-resolution and de-noising.	• A small training dataset *; Small anatomical structures may be easily buried and invisible in low-resolution images.
Minnema [23] (2019)	The proposed deep learning algorithm allows us to accurately classify metal artifacts as background noise, and to segment teeth and bony structures.	• A small training dataset *; Lacking independent unseen testing data *; Potential bias in the overall accuracy of the gold standard segmentations *.
Miki [38] (2017)	The proposed deep learning algorithm to classify tooth types on CBCTs yielded a high performance. This can be effectively used for automated preparation of dental charts and might be useful in forensic identification.	• A small training dataset *; Unstable classification performance due to the analyzed levels of the cross-sectional tooth images and metal artifacts;
Ghazvinian Zanjani [24] (2019)	The proposed end-to-end deep learning framework for the segmentation of individual teeth and the gingiva from intraoral scans outperforms state-of-the-art networks.	• A small training dataset *; Ex-vivo data *; Lacking independent unseen testing data *;
Kim [45] (2020)	The proposed automated segmentation method for full arch intraoral scan data is as accurate as a manual segmentation method. This tool could efficiently facilitate the digital setup process in orthodontic treatment.	• Ex-vivo data *; Unable to automatically detect the occlusion area.
Lian [25] (2020)	The proposed end-to-end deep neural network to automatically label individual teeth on raw dental surfaces acquired by 3D intraoral scanners outperforms the state-of-the-art methods for 3D shape segmentation.	• A small training dataset *; Scans only containing the maxillary dental surfaces with the complete 14 teeth *; Failed to properly handle missing teeth and additional braces in challenging cases; Lacking independent unseen testing data *;
Liu [27] (2016)	The proposed machine learning algorithm based on face scanning patterns could support current clinical practice of the screening and diagnosis of ASD	• A small training dataset *; Lacking independent unseen testing data *; Several influencing factors, such as age-/culture-adapted face scanning patterns and the characteristics of the ASD patients should be considered when applying the model to classify children with ASD *.
Knoops [26] (2019)	The proposed model can automatically analyze facial shape features and provide patient-specific treatment plans from a 3D facial scan. This may benefit the clinical decision-making process and improve clinical understanding of face shape as a marker for plastic and reconstructive surgery.	• Lacking independent unseen testing data *

3D, three-dimensional; AI, artificial intelligence; ASD, autism spectrum disorder; CBCT, cone beam computed tomography; CT, computed tomography; CNN, convolutional neural network; ROI, region of interest; SjS, Sjögren's syndrome; * risk of bias.

5. Conclusions

The AI models described in the included studies exhibited various potential applications for 3D imaging in dental medicine, such as automated diagnosis of cystic lesions, localization of anatomical landmarks, and classification/segmentation of teeth (see details in Table 3). The performance of most of the proposed machine learning algorithms was considered satisfactory for clinical use, but with room for improvement. Currently, none of the algorithms described are commercially available. It is expected that the developed AI systems will be available as open-source for others to verify their findings and this will eventually lead to true impact in different dental settings. By such an approach, they will also be more easily accessible and potentially user-friendly for dental practitioners.

Up to date, most of the proposed machine learning algorithms were designed to address specific clinical issues in various fields of dental medicine. In the future, it is expected that various relevant algorithms would be integrated into one intelligent workflow system specifically designed for dental clinic use [47]. After input of the patient's demographic data, medical history, clinical findings, 2D/3D diagnostic images, and/or intraoral/facial scans, the system could automatically conduct an overall analysis of the patient. The gathered data might contribute to a better understanding of the health condition of the respective patient and the development of personalized dental medicine, and subsequently, an individualized diagnosis, recommendations for comprehensive interdisciplinary treatment plans, and prediction of the treatment outcome and follow-up. This information will be provided to assist dental practitioners in making evidence-based decisions for each individual based on a real-time up-to-date big database. Furthermore, the capability of deep learning to analyze the information in each pixel/voxel unit may help to detect early lesions or unhealthy conditions that cannot be readily seen by human eyes. The future goals of AI development in dental medicine can be expected to not only improve patient care and radiologist's work but also surpass human experts in achieving more timely diagnoses. Long working hours and uncomfortable work environments may affect the performance of radiologists, whereas a more consistent performance of AI systems can be achieved regardless of working hours and conditions.

It is worth noting that although the development of AI in healthcare is vigorously supported by world-leading medical and technological institutions, the current evidence of AI applications for 3D imaging in dental medicine is very limited. The lack of adequate studies on this topic has resulted in the present methodological approach to provide findings from the literature rather than a pure systematic review. Thus, a selection bias could very likely not be eliminated due to the design of the study, which is certainly a relevant limitation of the present article. Nevertheless, the results presented might have a positive and stimulating impact on future studies and research in this field and hopefully will result in academic debate.

Author Contributions: Conceptualization, M.M.B.; Methodology, A.W.K.Y. and K.H.; Writing—Original Draft Preparation, K.H. and M.M.B.; Writing—Review and Editing, A.W.K.Y. and R.T.; Supervision, M.M.B.; Project Administration, M.M.B. All authors have read and agreed to the published version of the manuscript.

Funding: This research received no external funding.

Conflicts of Interest: The authors declare no conflict of interest.

References

1. Stone, P.; Brooks, R.; Brynjolfsson, E.; Calo, R.; Etzioni, O.; Hager, G.; Hirschberg, J.; Kalyanakrishnan, S.; Kamar, E.; Kraus, S.; et al. Artificial Intelligence and Life in 2030. One Hundred Year Study on Artificial Intelligence: Report of the 2015–2016 Study Panel, Stanford University, Stanford, CA. Available online: https://ai100.stanford.edu/2016-report (accessed on 12 March 2020).
2. Gandomi, A.; Haider, M. Beyond the hype: Big data concepts, methods, and analytics. *Int. J. Inf. Manag.* **2015**, *35*, 137–144. [CrossRef]
3. Jiang, F.; Jiang, Y.; Zhi, H.; Dong, Y.; Li, H.; Ma, S.; Wang, Y.; Dong, Q.; Shen, H.; Wang, Y. Artificial intelligence in healthcare: Past, present and future. *Stroke Vasc. Neurol.* **2017**, *2*, 230–243. [CrossRef] [PubMed]

4. Hamet, P.; Tremblay, J. Artificial intelligence in medicine. *Metabolism* **2017**, *69*, S36–S40. [CrossRef] [PubMed]
5. Fazal, M.I.; Patel, M.E.; Tye, J.; Gupta, Y. The past, present and future role of artificial intelligence in imaging. *Eur. J. Radiol.* **2018**, *105*, 246–250. [CrossRef] [PubMed]
6. Ferizi, U.; Besser, H.; Hysi, P.; Jacobs, J.; Rajapakse, C.S.; Chen, C.; Saha, P.K.; Honig, S.; Chang, G. Artificial intelligence applied to osteoporosis: A performance comparison of machine learning algorithms in predicting fragility fractures from MRI data. *J. Magn. Reson. Imaging* **2019**, *49*, 1029–1038. [CrossRef] [PubMed]
7. Schuhbaeck, A.; Otaki, Y.; Achenbach, S.; Schneider, C.; Slomka, P.; Berman, D.S.; Dey, D. Coronary calcium scoring from contrast coronary CT angiography using a semiautomated standardized method. *J. Cardiovasc. Comput. Tomogr.* **2015**, *9*, 446–453. [CrossRef]
8. Esteva, A.; Kuprel, B.; Novoa, R.A.; Ko, J.; Swetter, S.M.; Blau, H.M.; Thrun, S. Dermatologist-level classification of skin cancer with deep neural networks. *Nature* **2017**, *542*, 115–118. [CrossRef]
9. Litjens, G.; Kooi, T.; Bejnordi, B.E.; Setio, A.A.A.; Ciompi, F.; Ghafoorian, M.; van der Laak, J.; van Ginneken, B.; Sánchez, C.I. A survey on deep learning in medical image analysis. *Med. Image Anal.* **2017**, *42*, 60–88. [CrossRef]
10. Hosny, A.; Parmar, C.; Quackenbush, J.; Schwartz, L.H.; Aerts, H.J.W.L. Artificial intelligence in radiology. *Nat. Rev. Cancer* **2018**, *18*, 500–510. [CrossRef]
11. Hung, K.; Montalvao, C.; Tanaka, R.; Kawai, T.; Bornstein, M.M. The use and performance of artificial intelligence applications in dental and maxillofacial radiology: A systematic review. *Dentomaxillofac. Radiol.* **2020**, *49*, 20190107. [CrossRef]
12. Leite, A.F.; Vasconcelos, K.F.; Willems, H.; Jacobs, R. Radiomics and machine learning in oral healthcare. *Proteom. Clin. Appl.* **2020**, *14*, e1900040. [CrossRef] [PubMed]
13. Pauwels, R.; Araki, K.; Siewerdsen, J.H.; Thongvigitmanee, S.S. Technical aspects of dental CBCT: State of the art. *Dentomaxillofac. Radiol.* **2015**, *44*, 20140224. [CrossRef] [PubMed]
14. Baysal, A.; Sahan, A.O.; Ozturk, M.A.; Uysal, T. Reproducibility and reliability of three-dimensional soft tissue landmark identification using three-dimensional stereophotogrammetry. *Angle Orthod.* **2016**, *86*, 1004–1009. [CrossRef] [PubMed]
15. Hwang, J.J.; Jung, Y.H.; Cho, B.H.; Heo, M.S. An overview of deep learning in the field of dentistry. *Imaging Sci. Dent.* **2019**, *49*, 1–7. [CrossRef]
16. Okada, K.; Rysavy, S.; Flores, A.; Linguraru, M.G. Noninvasive differential diagnosis of dental periapical lesions in cone-beam CT scans. *Med. Phys.* **2015**, *42*, 1653–1665. [CrossRef]
17. Abdolali, F.; Zoroofi, R.A.; Otake, Y.; Sato, Y. Automated classification of maxillofacial cysts in cone beam CT images using contourlet transformation and Spherical Harmonics. *Comput. Methods Programs Biomed.* **2017**, *139*, 197–207. [CrossRef]
18. Yilmaz, E.; Kayikcioglu, T.; Kayipmaz, S. Computer-aided diagnosis of periapical cyst and keratocystic odontogenic tumor on cone beam computed tomography. *Comput. Methods Programs Biomed.* **2017**, *146*, 91–100. [CrossRef]
19. Lee, J.H.; Kim, D.H.; Jeong, S.N. Diagnosis of cystic lesions using panoramic and cone beam computed tomographic images based on deep learning neural network. *Oral Dis.* **2020**, *26*, 152–158. [CrossRef]
20. Ariji, Y.; Fukuda, M.; Kise, Y.; Nozawa, M.; Yanashita, Y.; Fujita, H.; Katsumata, A.; Ariji, E. Contrast-enhanced computed tomography image assessment of cervical lymph node metastasis in patients with oral cancer by using a deep learning system of artificial intelligence. *Oral Surg. Oral Med. Oral Pathol. Oral Radiol.* **2019**, *127*, 458–463. [CrossRef]
21. Montufar, J.; Romero, M.; Scougall-Vilchis, R.J. Automatic 3-dimensional cephalometric landmarking based on active shape models in related projections. *Am. J. Orthod. Dentofac. Orthop.* **2018**, *153*, 449–458. [CrossRef]
22. Montufar, J.; Romero, M.; Scougall-Vilchis, R.J. Hybrid approach for automatic cephalometric landmark annotation on cone-beam computed tomography volumes. *Am. J. Orthod. Dentofac. Orthop.* **2018**, *154*, 140–150. [CrossRef] [PubMed]
23. Minnema, J.; van Eijnatten, M.; Hendriksen, A.A.; Liberton, N.; Pelt, D.M.; Batenburg, K.J.; Forouzanfar, T.; Wolff, J. Segmentation of dental cone-beam CT scans affected by metal artifacts using a mixed-scale dense convolutional neural network. *Med. Phys.* **2019**, *46*, 5027–5035. [CrossRef] [PubMed]
24. Ghazvinian Zanjani, F.; Anssari Moin, D.; Verheij, B.; Claessen, F.; Cherici, T.; Tan, T.; de With, P.H.N. Deep learning approach to semantic segmentation in 3D point cloud intra-oral scans of teeth. *MIDL* **2019**, *102*, 557–571.

25. Lian, C.; Wang, L.; Wu, T.H.; Wang, F.; Yap, P.T.; Ko, C.C.; Shen, D. Deep multi-scale mesh feature learning for automated labeling of raw dental surfaces from 3D intraoral scanners. *IEEE Trans. Med. Imaging* **2020**, in press. [CrossRef]
26. Knoops, P.G.M.; Papaioannou, A.; Borghi, A.; Breakey, R.W.F.; Wilson, A.T.; Jeelani, O.; Zafeiriou, S.; Steinbacher, D.; Padwa, B.L.; Dunaway, D.J.; et al. A machine learning framework for automated diagnosis and computer-assisted planning in plastic and reconstructive surgery. *Sci. Rep.* **2019**, *9*, 13597. [CrossRef]
27. Liu, W.; Li, M.; Yi, L. Identifying children with autism spectrum disorder based on their face processing abnormality: A machine learning framework. *Autism Res.* **2016**, *9*, 888–998. [CrossRef]
28. Orhan, K.; Bayrakdar, I.S.; Ezhov, M.; Kravtsov, A.; Ozyurek, T. Evaluation of artificial intelligence for detecting periapical pathosis on cone-beam computed tomography scans. *Int. Endod. J.* **2020**, *53*, 680–689. [CrossRef]
29. Abdolali, F.; Zoroofi, R.A.; Otake, Y.; Sato, Y. A novel image-based retrieval system for characterization of maxillofacial lesions in cone beam CT images. *Int. J. Comput. Assist. Radiol. Surg.* **2019**, *14*, 785–796. [CrossRef]
30. Johari, M.; Esmaeili, F.; Andalib, A.; Garjani, S.; Saberkari, H. Detection of vertical root fractures in intact and endodontically treated premolar teeth by designing a probabilistic neural network: An ex vivo study. *Dentomaxillofac. Radiol.* **2017**, *46*, 20160107. [CrossRef]
31. Kann, B.H.; Aneja, S.; Loganadane, G.V.; Kelly, J.R.; Smith, S.M.; Decker, R.H.; Yu, J.B.; Park, H.S.; Yarbrough, W.G.; Malhotra, A.; et al. Pretreatment identification of head and neck cancer nodal metastasis and extranodal extension using deep learning neural networks. *Sci. Rep.* **2018**, *8*, 14036. [CrossRef]
32. Kise, Y.; Ikeda, H.; Fujii, T.; Fukuda, M.; Ariji, Y.; Fujita, H.; Katsumata, A.; Ariji, E. Preliminary study on the application of deep learning system to diagnosis of Sjögren's syndrome on CT images. *Dentomaxillofac. Radiol.* **2019**, *48*, 20190019. [CrossRef] [PubMed]
33. Cheng, E.; Chen, J.; Yang, J.; Deng, H.; Wu, Y.; Megalooikonomou, V.; Gable, B.; Ling, H. Automatic Dent-landmark detection in 3-D CBCT dental volumes. *Conf. Proc. IEEE Eng. Med. Biol. Soc.* **2011**, *2011*, 6204–6207. [PubMed]
34. Shahidi, S.; Bahrampour, E.; Soltanimehr, E.; Zamani, A.; Oshagh, M.; Moattari, M.; Mehdizadeh, A. The accuracy of a designed software for automated localization of craniofacial landmarks on CBCT images. *BMC Med. Imaging* **2014**, *14*, 32. [CrossRef] [PubMed]
35. Torosdagli, N.; Liberton, D.K.; Verma, P.; Sincan, M.; Lee, J.S.; Bagci, U. Deep geodesic learning for segmentation and anatomical landmarking. *IEEE Trans. Med. Imaging* **2019**, *38*, 919–931. [CrossRef] [PubMed]
36. Park, J.; Hwang, D.; Kim, K.Y.; Kang, S.K.; Kim, Y.K.; Lee, J.S. Computed tomography super-resolution using deep convolutional neural network. *Phys. Med. Biol.* **2018**, *63*, 145011. [CrossRef]
37. ter Haar Romeny, B.M. A deeper understanding of deep learning. In *Artificial Intelligence in Medical Imaging: Opportunities, Applications and Risks*, 1st ed.; Ranschaert, E.R., Morozov, S., Algra, P.R., Eds.; Springer: Berlin, Germany, 2019; pp. 25–38.
38. Miki, Y.; Muramatsu, C.; Hayashi, T.; Zhou, X.; Hara, T.; Katsumata, A.; Fujita, H. Classification of teeth in cone-beam CT using deep convolutional neural network. *Comput. Biol. Med.* **2017**, *80*, 24–29. [CrossRef]
39. Abdolali, F.; Zoroofi, R.A.; Otake, Y.; Sato, Y. Automatic segmentation of maxillofacial cysts in cone beam CT images. *Comput. Biol. Med.* **2016**, *72*, 108–119. [CrossRef]
40. Scarfe, W.C.; Azevedo, B.; Toghyani, S.; Farman, A.G. Cone beam computed tomographic imaging in orthodontics. *Aust. Dent. J.* **2017**, *62*, 33–50. [CrossRef]
41. Bornstein, M.M.; Yeung, W.K.A.; Montalvao, C.; Colsoul, N.; Parker, Q.A.; Jacobs, R. Facts and Fallacies of Radiation Risk in Dental Radiology. Available online: http://facdent.hku.hk/docs/ke/2019_Radiology_KE_booklet_en.pdf (accessed on 12 March 2020).
42. Yeung, A.W.K.; Jacobs, R.; Bornstein, M.M. Novel low-dose protocols using cone beam computed tomography in dental medicine: A review focusing on indications, limitations, and future possibilities. *Clin. Oral Investig.* **2019**, *23*, 2573–2581. [CrossRef]
43. Tuzoff, D.V.; Tuzova, L.N.; Bornstein, M.M.; Krasnov, A.S.; Kharchenko, M.A.; Nikolenko, S.I.; Sveshnikov, M.M.; Bednenko, G.B. Tooth detection and numbering in panoramic radiographs using convolutional neural networks. *Dentomaxillofac. Radiol.* **2019**, *48*, 20180051. [CrossRef]

44. Tomita, Y.; Uechi, J.; Konno, M.; Sasamoto, S.; Iijima, M.; Mizoguchi, I. Accuracy of digital models generated by conventional impression/plaster-model methods and intraoral scanning. *Dent. Mater. J.* **2018**, *37*, 628–633. [CrossRef] [PubMed]
45. Kim, T.; Cho, Y.; Kim, D.; Chang, M.; Kim, Y.J. Tooth segmentation of 3D scan data using generative adversarial networks. *Appl. Sci.* **2020**, *10*, 490. [CrossRef]
46. Morey, J.M.; Haney, N.M.; Kim, W. Applications of AI beyond image interpretation. In *Artificial Intelligence in Medical Imaging: Opportunities, Applications and Risks*, 1st ed.; Ranschaert, E.R., Morozov, S., Algra, P.R., Eds.; Springer: Berlin, Germany, 2019; pp. 129–144.
47. Chen, Y.W.; Stanley, K.; Att, W. Artificial intelligence in dentistry: Current applications and future perspectives. *Quintessence Int.* **2020**, *51*, 248–257. [PubMed]

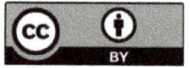

© 2020 by the authors. Licensee MDPI, Basel, Switzerland. This article is an open access article distributed under the terms and conditions of the Creative Commons Attribution (CC BY) license (http://creativecommons.org/licenses/by/4.0/).

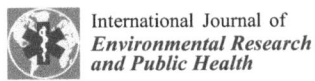

Article

Does Last Year's Cost Predict the Present Cost? An Application of Machine Leaning for the Japanese Area-Basis Public Health Insurance Database

Yoshiaki Nomura [1,*], Yoshimasa Ishii [2], Yota Chiba [2], Shunsuke Suzuki [2], Akira Suzuki [2], Senichi Suzuki [2], Kenji Morita [2], Joji Tanabe [2], Koji Yamakawa [2], Yasuo Ishiwata [2], Meu Ishikawa [1], Kaoru Sogabe [1], Erika Kakuta [3], Ayako Okada [4], Ryoko Otsuka [1] and Nobuhiro Hanada [1]

[1] Department of Translational Research, Tsurumi University School of Dental Medicine, Yokohama 230-8501, Japan; ishikawa-me@tsurumi-u.ac.jp (M.I.); sogabe-k@tsurumi-u.ac.jp (K.S.); otsuka-ryoko@tsurumi-u.ac.jp (R.O.); hanada-n@tsurumi-u.ac.jp (N.H.)

[2] Ebina Dental Association, Kanagawa 243-0421, Japan; ishiiryo141@gmail.com (Y.I.); yota@db3.so-net.ne.jp (Y.C.); shun-s@wg8.so-net.ne.jp (S.S.); suzuki@bell-dental.com (A.S.); lion@kd5.so-net.ne.jp (S.S.); morita-d-c-2@t06.itscom.net (K.M.); tanabedental5@me.com (J.T.); cherry@cherry-dental.com (K.Y.); yasuo-i@rb3.so-net.ne.jp (Y.I.)

[3] Department of Oral Microbiology, Tsurumi University School of Dental Medicine, Yokohama 230-8501, Japan; kakuta-erika@tsurumi-u.ac.jp

[4] Department of Operative Dentistry, Tsurumi University School of Dental Medicine, Yokohama 230-8501, Japan; okada-a@tsurumi-u.ac.jp

* Correspondence: nomura-y@tsurumi-u.ac.jp

Received: 14 November 2020; Accepted: 7 January 2021; Published: 12 January 2021

Abstract: The increasing healthcare cost imposes a large economic burden for the Japanese government. Predicting the healthcare cost may be a useful tool for policy making. A database of the area-basis public health insurance of one city was analyzed to predict the medical healthcare cost by the dental healthcare cost with a machine learning strategy. The 30,340 subjects who had continued registration of the area-basis public health insurance of Ebina city during April 2017 to September 2018 were analyzed. The sum of the healthcare cost was JPY 13,548,831,930. The per capita healthcare cost was JPY 446,567. The proportion of medical healthcare cost, medication cost, and dental healthcare cost was 78%, 15%, and 7%, respectively. By the results of the neural network model, the medical healthcare cost proportionally depended on the medical healthcare cost of the previous year. The dental healthcare cost of the previous year had a reducing effect on the medical healthcare cost. However, the effect was very small. Oral health may be a risk for chronic diseases. However, when evaluated by the healthcare cost, its effect was very small during the observation period.

Keywords: healthcare cost; medical healthcare cost; dental healthcare cost; zero-inflated model; neural network

1. Introduction

The increasing healthcare cost imposes a large economic burden for the Japanese government. In Japan, the national insurance system covers a wide range of treatment of diseases and injuries including dental treatment and medication. By the annual report of "Estimates of National Medical Care Expenditure, FY 2017", which summarizes the expense of the national health insurance, the total healthcare cost was

JPY 43.0710 trillion with a 2.2% increase on the previous fiscal year. It occupied 7.78% of the GDP and 10.66% of the national income. The per capita cost was JPY 339,900. Twenty-five percent of the source funding was from the national treasury and 13% from local governments [1].

Oral diseases are the most prevalent diseases globally and have serious health and economic burdens. The most frequent disease leading to death worldwide is a non-communicable disease. Oral health, especially the periodontal condition has been suggested to be affected by noncommunicable diseases [2–11]. An imbalance towards a periodontal immune response is underlined for other chronic diseases [11]. Epidemiological studies had shown that periodontitis was associated with the metabolic syndrome [3] and cardiovascular disease [4,7]. The suboptimal oral function was a potential risk of mortality [12,13]. Periodontitis was associated with an increased risk of all-cause mortality, mortality due to cardiovascular diseases, cancer, coronary heart disease, and cerebrovascular diseases [2]. The prevention and intervention of oral disease may lead to improving the health status and is finally expected to lead to reducing the medical healthcare cost.

In the previous report, statistical models were constructed to predict the healthcare cost by the periodontal status and dental healthcare cost [14,15]. The limitation of these studies were a small sample size and the subjects analyzed in these studies were adults who engaged in a specific occupation: High school teachers [14] and the clerk of the insurance company [15].

In contrast to previous studies, the area-basis public health insurance database contains a large sample size and subjects and their families engaged in a variety of occupations. By analyzing the area-basis public health insurance database, a more validated and general statistical model to evaluate the effect of oral health on the healthcare cost can be constructed.

In this study, a database of the area-basis public health insurance of one city was analyzed. The aim of this study was to present the descriptive statistics of the healthcare cost and to predict the medical healthcare cost by the dental healthcare cost.

2. Materials and Methods

2.1. Setting

Ebina city is located in Kanagawa Prefecture next to Tokyo, Capital of Japan. The population of Ebina city was 135,619 at 1 October 2020. Ninety-one subjects were born and 84 died during October 2020. Four hundred and seventy-two subjects were moved in and 440 subjects were moved out during October 2019. A total of 36,856 subjects were subscribed to the area-basis public health insurance of Ebina city at 1 April 2017 [16].

2.2. Database

The Japan Federation of National Health Insurance Organization constructed and provided the database software for all the cities or villages that managed the area-basis public health insurance. This database is called the Kokuho database. The abbreviation of "Koku" means nation and "ho" means insurance. This database is conventionally known as KDB. KDB summarizes the monthly healthcare cost per capita. Healthcare costs are summarized by the medical healthcare cost, medication cost, and dental healthcare cost. The medical healthcare cost was summarized separately by the hospitalized patients care cost and outpatients care cost. The data from April 2017 to September 2018 were completed in October 2020. In this study, the data during this duration were analyzed by the exported CSV file.

2.3. Statistical Modeling

2.3.1. Generalized Linear Model and Zero-Inflated Model

Before the application of the zero-inflated model, the medical and dental costs were categorized. Optimal categorizations were performed by the SPSS Statistics version 24.0 (IBM, Tokyo, Japan).

For the prediction of the medical healthcare cost, the generalized linear model and zero-inflated models were constructed [17]. The categorized medical healthcare cost was used as a dependent variable. The age, sex, categorized medical healthcare cost of the previous year, and the categorized dental healthcare cost of the previous year were used as an independent variable. The model fit was evaluated by Akaike's information criteria (AIC). To improve the model fit, link functions and distributions were changed. The model that had the least AIC was selected. The R software version 3.50 with AER, glm2, pscl, and MASS package was used.

2.3.2. Neural Network Model

The multilayer perceptron was applied to predict the medical healthcare cost [14,15,18]. The age, sex, medical healthcare cost of the previous year, and dental healthcare cost of the previous year were used as predictor values. The data were randomly divided into 15 groups. One group was used for the construction of the model and the model was trained by the other data of the 14 groups. The model construction and prediction were performed by the SPSS Modeler version 18.22 (IBM, Tokyo, Japan).

2.3.3. Support Vector Machine Regression

Support vector machine regression was performed by the R software with e1071 and the kernlab package. The model was constructed by the spline kernel as a kernel function. A four times-fold cross validation on the training data were used for training the model.

2.3.4. Generalized Boosted Regression Models

Generalized boosted regression models were constructed by the R software with the gbm package and the following parameter settings: Distribution = "gaussian", n.trees = 100, shrinkage = 0.1, interaction.depth = 3, bag.fraction = 0.5, train.fraction = 0.5, n.minobsinnode = 10, cv.folds = 5.

2.4. Ethics

The study protocol was approved by the Ethical Committee of Tsurumi University School of Dental Medicine (approval number: 1747).

3. Results

3.1. Descriptive Statistics of the Healthcare Cost

From April 2017 to September 2018, 6526 subjects were resigned from the area-basis national health insurance of Ebina city and 2901 subjects were newly affiliated. A total of JPY 14,899,646,550 were used as the healthcare cost during this period. The 30,340 subjects who had continued registration of the area-basis public health insurance of Ebina city were analyzed. The study population consisted of 15,787 men and 14,553 women, and their age was 53.23 +/− 19.60 for the mean and standard deviation, and 62 (41–69) for the median and 25th to 75th percentile. The healthcare cost of these subjects were JPY 13,548,831,930. The per capita healthcare cost was JPY 446,567. The itemized healthcare cost is shown in Figure 1. The medical healthcare cost, which is the sum of hospitalized patients care cost and outpatients care cost, was 78%

of the total cost and the dental healthcare cost was 7%. The itemized healthcare cost by the age groups was shown in Table S1. The distribution of the healthcare cost was skewed. During this one year and half period, 5707 (18.8%) subjects did not use a medical service, and 10,336 (34.1%) did not use a medication service, and 14,717 (48.5%) did not used a dental service.

The numbers indicate the sum of each cost during 2017 to the first half of 2018 (Japanese yen). The medical healthcare cost is the sum of hospitalized patients care cost and outpatient care cost. The itemized national healthcare cost was JPY 4,531,692,560 (37.6%) for the hospitalized patients care cost, JPY 5,992,460,680 (33.9%) for the outpatients' care cost, JPY 2,047,271,910 (18.1%) for the medication cost, and JPY 977,406,780 (6.7%) for the dental healthcare cost. The proportion of the itemized healthcare cost was not statistically significant when compared with the proportion of the national healthcare cost by the chi-square test ($p = 0.630$).

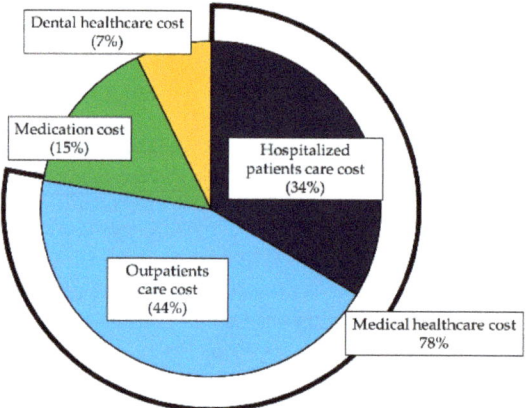

Figure 1. Total healthcare cost during 2017 to the first half of 2018.

3.2. Healthcare Cost by Specific Diseases

The KDB database contained a diagnosis of major diseases. For these diseases, the total healthcare cost during one year and half and the healthcare cost per capita were illustrated by a bar chart (Figure 2). For the total healthcare cost, musculoskeletal disease was highest followed by hypertension. For the healthcare cost per capita, peritoneal dialysis was highest followed by hemodialysis. However, the number of patients with peritoneal dialysis and hemodialysis were a very small fraction.

Int. J. Environ. Res. Public Health **2021**, *18*, 565

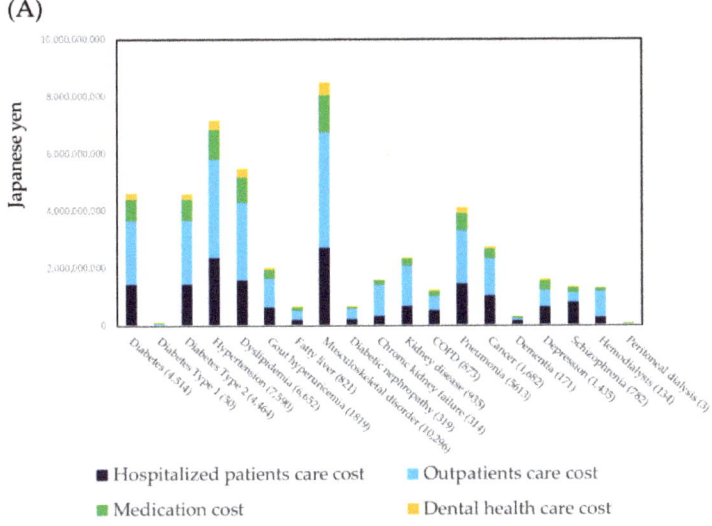

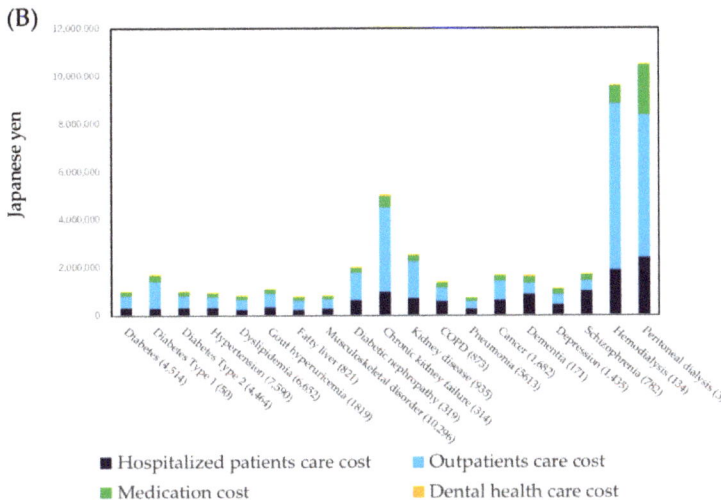

Figure 2. Healthcare cost of specific diseases. (**A**) Total healthcare cost, (**B**) healthcare cost per subjects.

The KDB database contained a diagnosis of major diseases and injuries. The healthcare cost by a specific disease was summarized by the sum of the healthcare cost during a one and half year period (A) and per capita during a one and a half year period (B).

3.3. Prediction of Medical Healthcare Cost

3.3.1. Descriptive Analysis

The scatter plot of medical cost against the medical cost of the previous year and dental cost of the previous year were shown in Figure 3. Plots were aggregated on the x and y axis. The regression lines by simple regression were not reliable. Therefore, to estimate the medical cost by the medical cost or dental cost of the previous year, statistical modeling is indispensable.

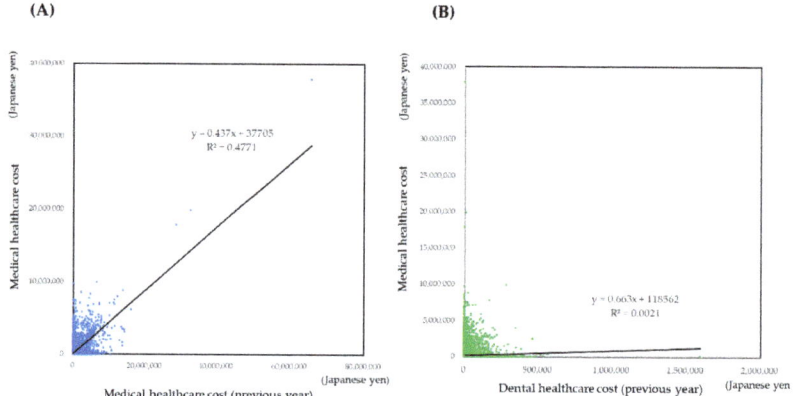

Figure 3. Cont.

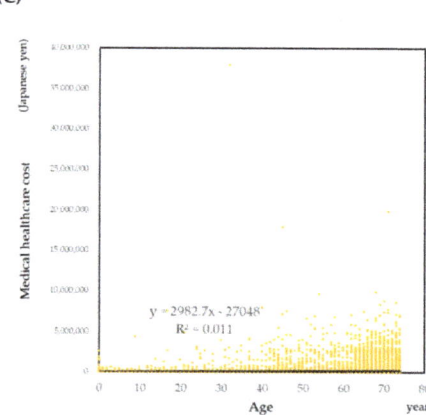

Figure 3. Scatter plot of medical healthcare cost against the medical healthcare cost of the previous year (**A**), dental healthcare cost of the previous year (**B**), and age (**C**). Plots were aggregated on the x or y axis.

3.3.2. Prediction of Medical Healthcare Cost by Regression Models

The medical healthcare cost during the half year was estimated by the regression model. The age, sex, medical healthcare cost of the previous year, and dental healthcare cost of the previous year were used as an independent variable. The conventional generalized linear model and zero-inflated model were applied (Table 1). When compared by Akaike's information criteria, the fittest model was the zero-inflated model. The zero-inflated model consisted of two components: Zero-inflation model and count model. For the zero-inflation model, the coefficient of the medical healthcare cost and dental healthcare cost of the previous year were negative and statistically significant. It indicated that subjects who used the medical or dental healthcare cost of the previous year tended not to use the medical healthcare cost the next year. By the count model, the coefficient of medical healthcare cost was positive and statistically significant. It indicated that the amount of the medical healthcare cost positively depended on the amount of the medical healthcare cost of the previous year. The coefficient of the dental healthcare cost was not statistically significant. It indicated that the amount of the medical healthcare cost was not dependent on the amount of dental healthcare cost of the previous year. For the prediction of the medical healthcare cost, the zero-inflated model gave us significant factors. However, there is a limitation for the zero-inflated model. Variables need to be treated as discrete variables.

3.3.3. Prediction of Medical Healthcare Cost by the Neural Network Model, Support Vector Machine Regression, and Generalized Boosted Regression Modeling (GBM)

Since the zero-inflated model has limitations for high values, the neural network model, support vector machine regression, and generalized boosted regression modeling (GBM) were applied to predict the medical healthcare cost. The age, sex, medical healthcare cost, and dental healthcare cost of the previous year were used as independent variables. The constructed neural network model was shown in Figure 4. The errors of square sum were 6687 for the learning step and 5626 for the test step. The predictive performances of these models are shown by the scatter plot of predictive values against the observed value: Neural network model (Figure 5A), Support Vector Machine Regression Figure 5B), and GBM (Figure 5C). The response surface of the prediction of the medical healthcare cost is shown in Figure 6. The medical healthcare cost proportionally depended on the medical healthcare cost of the previous year. The dental healthcare cost of the previous year had a reducing effect on the medical healthcare cost. However, the effect was very small. The information of the support vector machine regression and generalized boosted modeling were shown in Table S2 and Figure S1.

Table 1. Results of the regression model to estimate the medical healthcare cost.

Independent Variable	Generalized Linear Model	Zero-Inflated Model Zero-Inflation Model (Binomial, Link: Log-log)	
		Estimate	p-Value
(Intercept)		0.736	<0.001
Age		−0.0002	0.737
Sex (Women/Men)		−0.140	<0.001
Medical healthcare cost of the previous year		−0.259	<0.001
Dental healthcare cost of the previous year		−0.265	<0.001

Table 1. Cont.

	Estimate	p-value	Count model (Poisson, link: Log) Estimate	p-value
(Intercept)	0.374	<0.001	1.390	<0.001
Age	0.004	<0.001	0.004	<0.001
Sex (Women/Men)	0.031	<0.001	−0.023	<0.001
Medical healthcare cost of the previous year	0.114	<0.001	0.058	<0.001
Dental healthcare cost of the previous year	0.077	<0.001	−0.003	0.462
AIC	178,481		130,725	

The zero-inflated model consisted of two components: For the hurdle model, zero hurdle model, and count model and for the zero-inflated model, zero-inflated model, and count model, respectively. The zero-hurdle model and zero-inflation model are models to estimate if the samples exceeded zero or not. The count model is a model to estimate if the optimal distribution of the samples exceeded zero. AIC: Akaike's information criteria, the smaller AIC indicate the well model fit. The AICs of the models were very high.

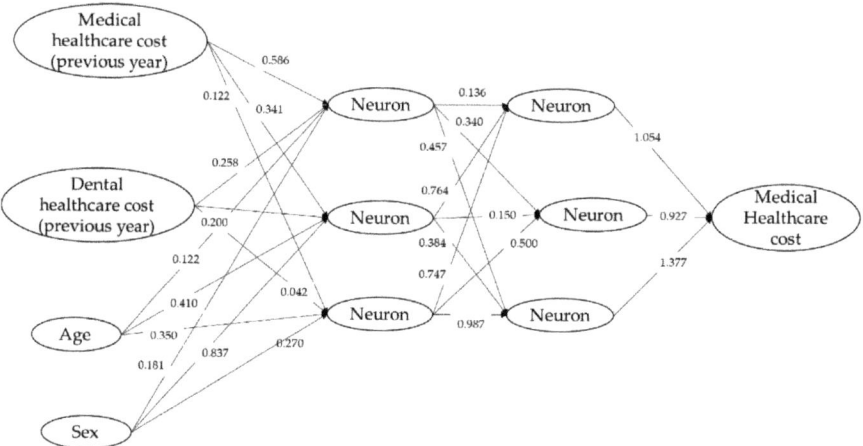

Figure 4. Neural network model for the prediction of medical healthcare cost.

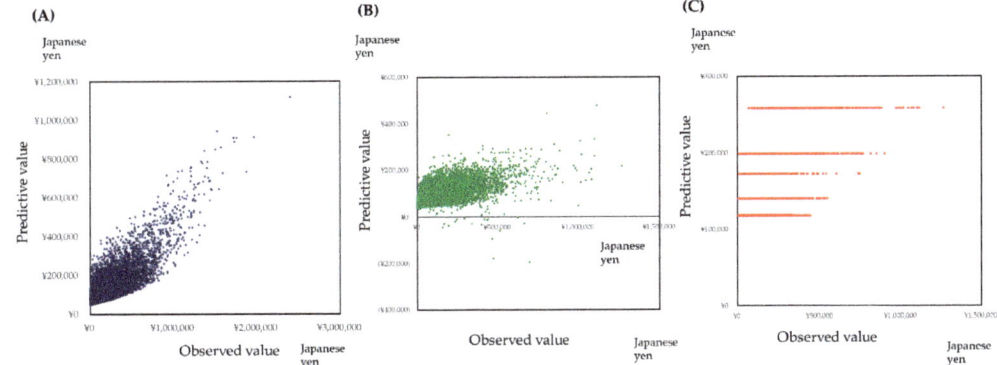

Figure 5. Predictive performance of the neural network model (**A**), support vector machine regression (**B**), and generalized boosted regression modeling (**C**). Predictive performance was shown by the scatter plot of the predictive value against the observed value.

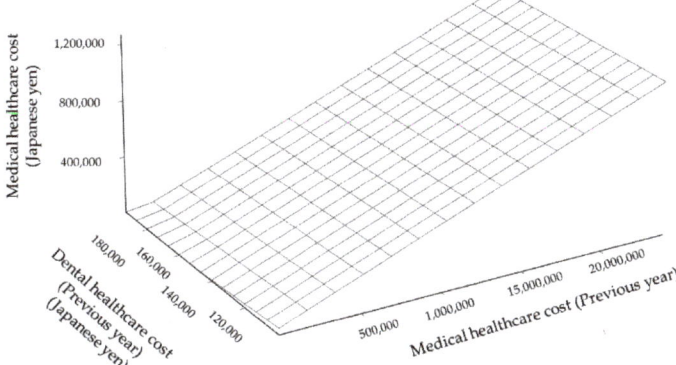

Figure 6. Response surface of the prediction of the medical healthcare cost by the medical healthcare cost of the previous year and dental healthcare cost of the previous year.

4. Discussion

The prediction of the healthcare cost is important for health policy making to decide the priority for the prevention of the disease. In this study, the medical healthcare cost was predicted by the medical healthcare cost of the previous year and the dental healthcare cost of the previous year. Our previous report had shown that conventional regression models were not applicable for the prediction of the medical cost [14,15].

The proportion of the itemized healthcare cost was not statistically significant when compared with the national healthcare cost. It indicated that the data analyzed in this study represented the national healthcare cost of Japan (Figure 1).

Some studies tried to predict the healthcare cost by the statistical modeling [19–24]. The age, gender, and a previous year's healthcare cost are strong predictors [24]. By the simulation presented in Figures 4 and 6, the medical healthcare cost increased with the increase of the previous year's medical healthcare cost. As shown in Figure 3, healthcare costs were aggregated on the x or y axis. It indicates that healthcare costs were abruptly consumed. One reason may derive from the subscribers' characteristics of the area-basis public health insurance. The proportion of low-income subscribers is higher than the other insurance [25]. In addition, the subscribers may not afford to spend the healthcare cost to maintain their health status.

As shown in Figure 2, about 1/3 of the subjects used the healthcare cost for musculoskeletal disorders. The number of subjects that used the healthcare cost for musculoskeletal disorders was higher than that of hypertension. In Japan, other than clinics of orthopedics, there are many treatment places managed by the bonesetter. These treatment places provide a massage, electric stimulation therapy, and hyperthermia treatment as rehabilitation. The national insurance system covers these treatments. It may be one of the reasons that many subjects used the healthcare cost for musculoskeletal disorders. The healthcare cost by kidney diseases was very high. More than JPY 10,000,000 per subject were used for the patients treated by hemodialysis. However, these patients were a tiny fraction. The prevention of kidney diseases by a high risk strategy may be a useful tool to reduce the healthcare cost.

There are many limitations to predict the healthcare cost by the conventional regression models. One of the solutions is to apply the zero-inflated model which consists of two components. However, this statistical model has a serious limitation. The variable that this model can deal with is a discrete variable. The neural network model can deal with both discrete and contentious variables. Our previous studies and the other study successfully predicted the medical healthcare cost by the neural network model [14,15,18]. Therefore, the neural network model as a nonlinear model may be an optimal statistical model to predict the healthcare cost.

When focusing on the axis of dental healthcare costs shown in Figure 6, spending the dental healthcare cost reduced the medical healthcare cost. However, its effect was a very tiny fraction. Periodontal disease was a risk for diabetes mellitus and diabetic complications: Diabetic retinopathy, neuropathy, nephropathy, cardiovascular complications, and mortality [26]. Oral health disorders were risks of hypertension [27]. The periodontal status affected hypertension [28]. Oral infections affected the prognosis of the patients with kidney disease [29,30]. The proportion of the medical healthcare cost of diabetes, hypertension, and kidney diseases was high (Figure 2A).

Poor oral hygiene has been suggested to be a risk for pneumonia, especially aspiration pneumonia [31]. Dental biofilm contains potential respiratory pathogens [32]. Oral hygiene behaviors including professional tooth cleaning by attending a dental clinic were associated with pneumonia [33]. Oral health intervention can reduce the incidence of pneumonia [34,35]. Therefore, using the dental healthcare cost is expected to reduce the healthcare cost for pneumonia. However, the study population of these studies were older adults. The subjects analyzed in this study were less than 75 years old. Insurance for the older adults over 75 years were different from the area-basis public health insurance. It is one of the limitations of this study. The prevalence of diseases and subsequent expenditure of healthcare cost may be different when limited to older adults. Older adults over the age of 65 spent four times the healthcare cost of the subjects less than 65 years old [1].

Improving the oral health status through dental treatment is expected to promote the health status and lead to the reduction of the medical healthcare cost. The Japanese insurance system covers not only the dental treatment, but also the supportive therapy by regular follow ups. However, when evaluating the health status by the medical healthcare cost, the dental treatment had an exiguous effect during a short period. The dental healthcare cost is low when compared to the medical healthcare costs. Oral health promotion affects the reducing prevalence of hypertension and type 2 diabetes, it will effectively act on reducing total healthcare costs. Therefore, a long term basis observational study is necessary to evaluate the effect of oral health on the medical healthcare cost. It is one of the limitations of this study. Electric data accumulation of the healthcare cost is just getting started in Japan.

5. Conclusions

The area-basis public health insurance database contains subjects with a wide range of age groups and their family members engaged in a variety of occupations. By analyzing this database, the robust statistical model for prediction can be obtained. Among the machine learning tools, the neural network model was the best method to predict the healthcare cost. The healthcare cost largely depended on the medical healthcare cost of the previous year. In addition, the dental treatment had an exiguous effect on the reduction of the medical healthcare cost.

Supplementary Materials: The following are available online at http://www.mdpi.com/1660-4601/18/2/565/s1. Figure S1: Relative influence of the factors for the medical healthcare cost by generalized boosted model; Table S1: Descriptive statistics of healthcare cost by age groups; Table S2: Information for the support vector machine regression model.

Author Contributions: Conceptualization, Y.N., Y.I. (Yoshimasa Ishii), S.S. (Shunsuke Suzuki), K.M., A.S., S.S. (Senichi Suzuki), J.T., Y.I. (Yasuo Ishiwata), K.Y., and Y.C.; methodology, Y.N., Y.I. (Yasuo Ishiwata), S.S. (Shunsuke Suzuki), K.M., A.S., S.S. (Senichi Suzuki), J.T., Y.I. (Yoshimasa Ishii), K.Y., and Y.C.; software, Y.N.; validation, Y.N. and Y.I. (Yoshimasa Ishii); formal analysis, Y.N.; investigation, Y.I. (Yoshimasa Ishii), S.S. (Shunsuke Suzuki), K.M., A.S., S.S. (Senichi Suzuki), J.T., Y.I. (Yasuo Ishiwata), K.Y., and Y.C.; data curation, M.I., K.S., E.K., A.O., and R.O.; writing—original draft preparation, Y.N.; writing—review and editing, Y.N.; visualization, Y.N.; project administration, Y.N., Y.I. (Yoshimasa Ishii), S.S. (Shunsuke Suzuki), K.M., A.S., S.S. (Senichi Suzuki), J.T., Y.I. (Yasuo Ishiwata), K.Y., and Y.C.; funding acquisition, S.S. (Senichi Suzuki), Y.I. (Yasuo Ishiwata), and N.H. All authors have read and agreed to the published version of the manuscript.

Funding: This research was funded by the annual budget of Ebina city for health promotion.

Institutional Review Board Statement: The study protocol was approved by the Ethical Committee of Tsurumi University School of Dental Medicine (approval number: 1747).

Informed Consent Statement: Not applicable.

Data Availability Statement: For the availability of data, approval of Ebina city council is necessary. If there is a reasonable reason, please ask the author Yoshimasa Ishii.

Acknowledgments: We thank Masaru Uchino, Mayor of Ebina city for adopting this project as a health promotion policy plan of Ebina city and the supporting funds.

Conflicts of Interest: The authors declare no conflict of interest.

References

1. Estimates of National Medical Care Expenditure, FY 2017. Available online: https://www.mhlw.go.jp/english/database/db-hss/enmce_2017.html (accessed on 14 October 2020).
2. Romandini, M.; Baima, G.; Antonoglou, G.; Bueno, J.; Figuero, E.; Sanz, M. Periodontitis, Edentulism, and Risk of Mortality: A Systematic Review with Meta-analyses. *J. Dent. Res.* **2020**. [CrossRef]
3. Gobin, R.; Tian, D.; Liu, Q.; Wang, J. Periodontal Diseases and the Risk of Metabolic Syndrome: An Updated Systematic Review and Meta-Analysis. *Front. Endocrinol.* **2020**, *11*, 336. [CrossRef] [PubMed]
4. Orlandi, M.; Graziani, F.; D'Aiuto, F. Periodontal therapy and cardiovascular risk. *Periodontology 2000* **2020**, *83*, 107–124. [CrossRef] [PubMed]
5. Jepsen, S.; Suvan, J.; Deschner, J. The association of periodontal diseases with metabolic syndrome and obesity. *Periodontology 2000* **2020**, *83*, 125–153. [CrossRef] [PubMed]
6. Genco, R.J.; Sanz, M. Clinical and public health implications of periodontal and systemic diseases: An overview. *Periodontology 2000* **2020**, *83*, 7–13. [CrossRef]
7. Sanz, M.; Castillo, M.D.A.; Jepsen, S.; Juanatey, G.J.R.; D'Aiuto, F.; Bouchard, P.; Chapple, I.; Dietrich, T.; Gotsman, I.; Graziani, F.; et al. Periodontitis and cardiovascular diseases: Consensus report. *J. Clin. Periodontol.* **2020**, *47*, 268–288. [CrossRef]

8. Bourgeois, D.; Inquimbert, C.; Ottolenghi, L.; Carrouel, F. Periodontal Pathogens as Risk Factors of Cardiovascular Diseases, Diabetes, Rheumatoid Arthritis, Cancer, and Chronic Obstructive Pulmonary Disease-Is There Cause for Consideration? *Microorganisms* **2019**, *7*, 424. [CrossRef]
9. Peres, M.A.; Macpherson, L.M.D.; Weyant, R.J.; Daly, B.; Venturelli, R.; Mathur, M.R.; Listl, S.; Celeste, R.K.; Herreño, G.C.C.; Kearns, C.; et al. Oral diseases: A global public health challenge. *Lancet* **2019**, *394*, 249–260. [CrossRef]
10. Sanz, M.; Ceriello, A.; Buysschaert, M.; Chapple, I.; Demmer, R.T.; Graziani, F.; Herrera, D.; Jepsen, S.; Lione, L.; Madianos, P.; et al. Scientific evidence on the links between periodontal diseases and diabetes: Consensus report and guidelines of the joint workshop on periodontal diseases and diabetes by the International Diabetes Federation and the European Federation of Periodontology. *J. Clin. Periodontol.* **2018**, *45*, 138–149. [CrossRef]
11. Cardoso, E.M.; Reis, C.; Céspedes, M.M.C. Chronic periodontitis, inflammatory cytokines, and interrelationship with other chronic diseases. *Postgrad. Med.* **2018**, *130*, 98–104. [CrossRef]
12. Nomura, Y.; Kakuta, E.; Okada, A.; Otsuka, R.; Shimada, M.; Tomizawa, Y.; Taguchi, C.; Arikawa, K.; Daikoku, H.; Sato, T.; et al. Impact of the Serum Level of Albumin and Self-Assessed Chewing Ability on Mortality, QOL, and ADLs for Community-Dwelling Older Adults at the Age of 85: A 15 Year Follow up Study. *Nutrients* **2020**, *12*, 3315. [CrossRef]
13. Nomura, Y.; Kakuta, E.; Okada, A.; Otsuka, R.; Shimada, M.; Tomizawa, Y.; Taguchi, C.; Arikawa, K.; Daikoku, H.; Sato, T.; et al. Effects of self-assessed chewing ability, tooth loss and serum albumin on mortality in 80-year-old individuals: A 20-year follow-up study. *BMC Oral Health* **2020**, *20*, 122. [CrossRef] [PubMed]
14. Kakuta, E.; Nomura, Y.; Naono, Y.; Koresawa, K.; Shimizu, K.; Hanada, N. Correlation between health-care costs and salivary tests. *Int. Dent. J.* **2013**, *63*, 249–253. [CrossRef] [PubMed]
15. Nomura, Y.; Sato, T.; Kamoshida, Y.; Suzuki, S.; Okada, A.; Otsuka, R.; Kakuta, E.; Hanada, N. Prediction of Health Care Costs by Dental Health Care Costs and Periodontal Status. *Appl. Sci.* **2020**, *10*, 3140. [CrossRef]
16. Ebina City Official Website. Available online: https://www.city.ebina.kanagawa.jp/shisei/denshi/toukei/jinko/1009539.html (accessed on 14 October 2020).
17. Nomura, Y.; Okada, A.; Kakuta, E.; Otsuka, R.; Saito, H.; Maekawa, H.; Daikoku, H.; Hanada, N.; Sato, T. Workforce and Contents of Home Dental Care in Japanese Insurance System. *Int. J. Dent.* **2020**, *2020*, 7316796. [CrossRef]
18. Otsuka, R.; Nomura, Y.; Okada, A.; Uematsu, H.; Nakano, M.; Hikiji, K.; Hanada, N.; Momoi, Y. Properties of manual toothbrush that influence on plaque removal of interproximal surface in vitro. *J. Dent. Sci.* **2020**, *15*, 14–21. [CrossRef]
19. Morid, M.A.; Sheng, O.R.L.; Kawamoto, K.; Ault, T.; Dorius, J.; Abdelrahman, S. Healthcare cost prediction: Leveraging fine-grain temporal patterns. *J. Biomed. Inform.* **2019**, *91*, 103113. [CrossRef]
20. Morid, M.A.; Sheng, O.R.L.; Kawamoto, K.; Abdelrahman, S. Learning hidden patterns from patient multivariate time series data using convolutional neural networks: A case study of healthcare cost prediction. *J. Biomed. Inform.* **2020**, *111*, 103565. [CrossRef]
21. Mazumdar, M.; Lin, J.-Y.J.; Zhang, W.; Li, L.; Liu, M.; Dharmarajan, K.V.; Sanderson, M.; Isola, L.; Hu, L. Comparison of statistical and machine learning models for healthcare cost data: A simulation study motivated by Oncology Care Model (OCM) data. *BMC Health Serv. Res.* **2020**, *20*, 350. [CrossRef]
22. Orueta, J.F.; Alvarez, G.A.; Aurrekoetxea, J.J.; Goñi, G.M. FINGER (Forming and Identifying New Groups of Expected Risks): Developing and validating a new predictive model to identify patients with high healthcare cost and at risk of admission. *BMJ Open* **2018**, *8*, e019830. [CrossRef]
23. Jones, A.M.; Lomas, J.; Rice, N. Healthcare Cost Regressions: Going Beyond the Mean to Estimate the Full Distribution. *Health Econ.* **2015**, *24*, 1192–1212. [CrossRef] [PubMed]
24. Otani, K.; Baden, W.W. Healthcare cost and predictive factors: High- and low-utilization model development. *Health Mark. Q.* **2009**, *26*, 198–208. [CrossRef] [PubMed]
25. Topics of Ministry Health, Labor and Welfare. Available online: https://www.mhlw.go.jp/topics/2012/02/dl/tp120205-1-13.pdf (accessed on 14 October 2020).

26. Nguyen, A.T.M.; Akhter, R.; Garde, S.; Scott, C.; Twigg, S.M.; Colagiuri, S.; Ajwani, S.; Eberhard, J. The association of periodontal disease with the complications of diabetes mellitus. A systematic review. *Diabetes Res. Clin. Pract.* **2020**, *165*, 108244. [CrossRef] [PubMed]
27. Iwashima, Y.; Kokubo, Y.; Ono, T.; Yoshimuta, Y.; Kida, M.; Kosaka, T.; Maeda, Y.; Kawano, Y.; Miyamoto, Y. Additive interaction of oral health disorders on risk of hypertension in a Japanese urban population: The Suita Study. *Am. J. Hypertens.* **2014**, *27*, 710–719. [CrossRef]
28. Nimma, V.; Talla, H.; Poosa, M.; Gopaladas, M.; Meesala, D.; Jayanth, L. Influence of Hypertension on pH of Saliva and Flow Rate in Elder Adults Correlating with Oral Health Status. *J. Clin. Diagn. Res.* **2016**, *10*, ZC34–ZC36. [CrossRef]
29. Sarmento, D.J.D.S.; Caliento, R.; Maciel, R.F.; Braz-Silva, P.H.; Pestana, J.O.M.D.A.; Lockhart, P.B.; Gallottini, M. Poor oral health status and short-term outcome of kidney transplantation. *Spec. Care Dent.* **2020**, *40*, 549–554. [CrossRef]
30. Wallace, K.; Shafique, S.; Piamjariyakul, U. The relationship between oral health and hemodialysis treatment among adults with chronic kidney disease: A systematic review. *Nephrol. Nurs. J.* **2019**, *46*, 375–394.
31. Nomura, Y.; Takei, N.; Ishii, T.; Takada, K.; Amitani, Y.; Koganezawa, H.; Fukuhara, S.; Asai, K.; Uozumi, R.; Bessho, K. Factors that affect oral care outcomes for institutionalized elderly. *Int. J. Dent.* **2018**, *2018*, 2478408. [CrossRef]
32. Scannapieco, F.A.; Shay, K. Oral health disparities in older adults: Oral bacteria, inflammation, and aspiration pneumonia. *Dent. Clin. North Am.* **2014**, *58*, 771–782. [CrossRef]
33. Son, M.; Jo, S.; Lee, J.S.; Lee, D.H. Association between oral health and incidence of pneumonia: A population-based cohort study from Korea. *Sci. Rep.* **2020**, *10*, 9576. [CrossRef]
34. Schwendicke, F.; Stolpe, M.; Müller, F. Professional oral health care for preventing nursing home-acquired pneumonia: A cost-effectiveness and value of information analysis. *J. Clin. Periodontol.* **2017**, *44*, 1236–1244. [CrossRef] [PubMed]
35. Haghighi, A.; Shafipour, V.; Nesami, B.M.; Baradari, G.A.; Charati, Y.J. The impact of oral care on oral health status and prevention of ventilator-associated pneumonia in critically ill patients. *Aust. Crit. Care* **2017**, *30*, 69–73. [CrossRef] [PubMed]

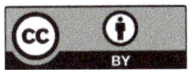

© 2021 by the authors. Licensee MDPI, Basel, Switzerland. This article is an open access article distributed under the terms and conditions of the Creative Commons Attribution (CC BY) license (http://creativecommons.org/licenses/by/4.0/).

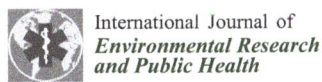

Review

Big Data and Digitalization in Dentistry: A Systematic Review of the Ethical Issues

Maddalena Favaretto [1],*, David Shaw [1], Eva De Clercq [1], Tim Joda [2] and Bernice Simone Elger [1]

1. Institute for Biomedical Ethics, University of Basel, 4056 Basel, Switzerland; david.shaw@unibas.ch (D.S.); eva.declercq@unibas.ch (E.D.C.); b.elger@unibas.ch (B.S.E.)
2. Department of Reconstructive Dentistry, University Center for Dental Medicine Basel, 4058 Basel, Switzerland; tim.joda@unibas.ch
* Correspondence: maddalena.favaretto@unibas.ch; Tel.: +416-1207-0203

Received: 11 March 2020; Accepted: 4 April 2020; Published: 6 April 2020

Abstract: Big Data and Internet and Communication Technologies (ICT) are being increasingly implemented in the healthcare sector. Similarly, research in the field of dental medicine is exploring the potential beneficial uses of digital data both for dental practice and in research. As digitalization is raising numerous novel and unpredictable ethical challenges in the biomedical context, our purpose in this study is to map the debate on the currently discussed ethical issues in digital dentistry through a systematic review of the literature. Four databases (Web of Science, Pub Med, Scopus, and Cinahl) were systematically searched. The study results highlight how most of the issues discussed by the retrieved literature are in line with the ethical challenges that digital technologies are introducing in healthcare such as privacy, anonymity, security, and informed consent. In addition, image forgery aimed at scientific misconduct and insurance fraud was frequently reported, together with issues of online professionalism and commercial interests sought through digital means.

Keywords: Big Data; digital dentistry; oral health; ethical issues

1. Introduction

The sophistication and increased use of Internet and Communication Technologies (ICT), the rise of Big Data and algorithmic analysis, and the origin of the Internet of Things (IOT) are a plethora of interconnected phenomena that is currently having an enormous impact on today's society and that is affecting almost all spheres of our lives. In recent years, we have seen an exponential growth in the generation, storage, and collection of computational data and the digital revolution is transforming an increasing number of sectors in our society [1,2].

In the biomedical context, for instance, digital technologies are finding numerous novel applications to improve healthcare, cut costs for hospitals, and maximize treatment effectiveness for patients. Examples of such implementations include the development of electronic health records (EHRs) and smarter hospitals for increased workflow [3], personalized medicine and linkage of health data [4], clinical decision support for novel treatment concepts [5], and deep learning and Artificial Intelligence (AI) for diagnostic analysis [6]. In addition, the implementation of mobile technologies into the medical sector is fundamentally altering the ways in which healthcare is perceived, delivered, and consumed. Thanks to the ubiquity of smartphones and wearable technologies, mobile health (mHealth) applications are currently being explored by healthcare providers and companies for remote measurement of health and provision of healthcare services [7].

Dentistry, as a branch of medicine, has not remained unaffected by the digital revolution. The trend in digitalization has led to an increased production of computer-generated data in a growing number of dental disciplines and fields—for example, oral and maxillofacial pathology and surgery, prosthodontics and implant dentistry, and oral public health [8–10]. For this reason, research in the field of dental medicine is currently focusing on exploring the numerous potential beneficial applications of digital and computer-generated data both for dental practice and in research. Population-based linkage of patient-level information could expand new approaches for research such as assisting with the identification of unknown correlations of oral diseases with suspected and new contributing factors and furthering the creation of new treatment concepts [11]. AI applications could help enhance the analysis of the relationship between prevention and treatment techniques in the field of oral health [12]. Digital imaging could promote accurate tracking of the distribution and prevalence of oral diseases to improve healthcare service provisions [13]. Finally, the creation of the digital or virtual dental patient, through the application of sophisticated dental imaging techniques (such as 3D con-beam computed tomography (CBCT) and 3D printed models) could be used for precise pre-operative clinical assessment and simulation of treatment planning in dental practice [9,14]. As these technologies are still at the early phases of implementation, technical issues and disadvantages might also emerge. For instance, data collection for the implementation of Big Data applications and AI must be done systematically according to harmonized and inter-linkable data standards, otherwise issues of data managing and garbage data accumulation might arise [15]. AI for diagnostic purposes is still in the very early phases, where its accuracy is being assessed, and although they are revealing themselves to be valuable for image-based diagnoses, analysis of diverse and massive EHR data still remains challenging [16]. Finally, with regards to the simulation of a 3D virtual dental patient, dataset superimposition techniques are still experimental and none of the currently available imaging techniques are sufficient to capture the complete dataset needed to create the 3D output in a single-step procedure [9].

In the past few years, alongside the ambitious promises of digital technologies in healthcare, the research community has also highlighted many of the potential ethical issues that Big Data and ICT are raising for both patients and other members of society. In the biomedical context, data technologies have been claimed to exacerbate issues of informed consent for both patients and research participants [17,18], and to create new issues regarding privacy, confidentiality [19–21], data security and data protection [22], and patient anonymization [23] and discrimination [24–26]. In addition, recent research has also emphasized additional pressing challenges that could emerge from the inattentive use of increasingly sophisticated digital technologies, such as issues of accuracy and accountability in the use of diagnostic algorithms [27] and the exacerbation of healthcare inequalities [25].

As dentistry is also undergoing the digital path, similar ethical issues might emerge from the application of ICT and Big Data technologies. To the best of our knowledge, there is currently no systematic evaluation of the different ethical issues raised by Big Data and ICT in the field of dentistry, as most of the literature on the topic generally focuses on non-dental medicine and healthcare [28]. As timely ethical evaluation is a consistent part of appropriate health technology assessment [29] and because recent literature has focused on the ethical issues concerning health-related Big Data [28], it is of the utmost importance to map the occurrence of the ethical issues related to the application of heterogeneous digital technologies in dental medicine and to investigate if specific ethical issues for dental Big Data are emerging.

We thus performed a systematic review of the literature. The study has the following aims: (1) mapping the identified ethical issues related to the digitalization of dental medicine and the applications of Big Data and ICT in oral healthcare; (2) investigating the suggested solutions proposed by the literature; and (3) understanding if some applications and practices in digital dentistry could also help overcome some ethical issues.

2. Materials and Methods

We performed a systematic literature review by searching four databases: PubMed, Web of Science, Scopus, and Cinahl. The following search terms were used: "big data", "digital data", "data linkage", "electronic health record *", "EHR", "digital *", "artificial intelligence", "data analytics", "information technology", "dentist *", "dental *", "oral health", "orthodont *", "ethic *", and "moral *". No restriction was placed on the type of methodology used in the paper (qualititative, qualitative, mixed methods, or theoretical). No time restriction was used. In order to enhance reproducibility of the study, we only included original research articles from peer-reviewed journals; therefore, grey literature, books (monographs and edited volumes), conference proceedings, dissertations, and posters were omitted. English was selected as it is the designated language of the highest number of peer-reviewed academic journals. The search was performed on 24 of January 2020 (see Table 1).

Table 1. Search terms.

No.	Match Search Terms	Pub Med	Web of Science	Scopus	Cinahl
1	("big data" OR "digital data" OR "data linkage" OR "electronic health record*" OR "EHR" OR "digital*" OR "artificial intelligence" OR "data analytics" OR "information technology")	251,004	4,682,526	1,750,766	67,116
2	("dentist*" OR "dental *" OR "oral health" OR "orthodont*")	827,547	1,409,796	613,348	158,231
3	("ethic *" OR "moral*")	334,537	582,299	528,738	98,246
4	1 AND 2 AND 3	190	186	71	63

We followed the protocol from the Preferred Reporting Item for Systematic Reviews and Meta-Analyses (PRISMA) method [30], which resulted in 510 papers. We scanned the results for duplicates (125) and 385 papers remained. In this phase, we included all articles that focused on digitalization of dentistry or on one specific digital technology in the field of dentistry and that mentioned, enumerated, discussed, or described one or more ethical challenge related to digitalization. Papers that only described a technology from a technical point of view, that did not focus on dentistry or focused generally on medical practice, or that did not relate to the ethical challenges of digitalization were excluded. Additional papers (27) were excluded because they were book sections, posters, conference proceedings, or not in English. In total, 356 papers were excluded.

We subsequently scanned the references of the remaining 29 articles to identify additional relevant studies. We added five papers through this process. The final sample included 34 articles. During the next phase, the first author read the full texts in their length. After thorough evaluation, eight articles were excluded for the following reasons: (1) they did not discuss or mention any ethical issue related to the technology discussed in the study; and (2) they did not refer to any digital implementation in dentistry (see Figure 1).

The subsequent phase of the study involved the analysis of the remaining 26 articles. Regarding data analysis, we carried out a narrative synthesis of included publications [31]. Therefore, we extracted the following information relevant to the aim of the present study and to the research question from the papers: year and country of publication; methodology; type of technology or digital application discussed; field of application of the article; ethical issues that emerge from the use of the technology; technical issues that might exacerbate the ethical issues discussed; suggested potential solutions to the issue(s); and ethical issues that the technology could help overcome.

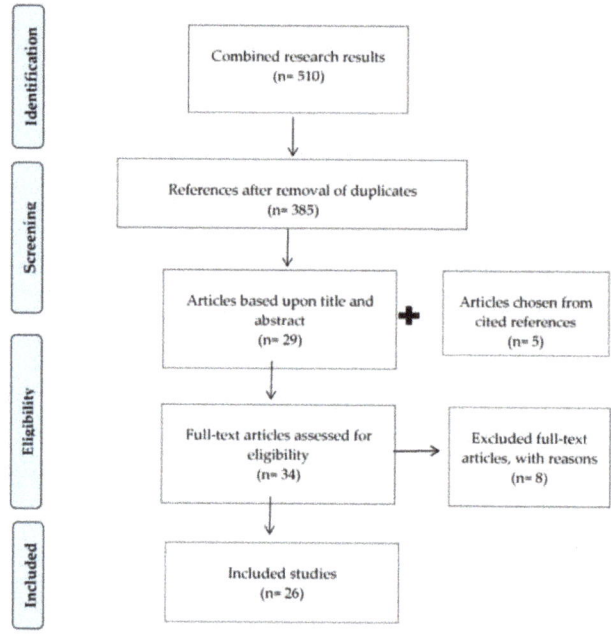

Figure 1. Preferred Reporting Item for Systematic Reviews and Meta-Analyses (PRISMA) flowchart.

3. Results

Among the 26 papers included in our analysis, 22 were theoretical papers that critically discussed the impact of digitalization in the field of dentistry or that discussed a specific technology highlighting its promises and some of its ethical challenges. Among the remaining papers, three applied empirical methods and one was a feasibility study. The majority of papers (n = 20) were published after 2010, five were published between 2008 and 2010, and one of them was from 1996. Half of the articles (n = 13) were from the United States, five came from the United Kingdom, and four from India. The remaining ones came from Belgium, Brazil, Germany, and South Africa. Regarding the type of technological application they discussed, almost one-third of the papers (n = 8) analyzed digital photography, radiology and computed imaging; six papers discussed the impact of digital communication and social media in dentistry; three articles focused on electronic health records (EHRs) and patient records; another three discussed the promises and challenges of mobile health and teledentistry; and an additional three records focused on data linkage and personalized medicine. In addition, two papers broadly discussed the challenges and promises of ICT and digital implementations in dentistry, while one paper focused on search engine optimizations in dental practices. Finally, concerning the field of application of the different papers, 10 articles discussed the ethical issues of digitalization regarding dental practice, nine discussed digitalization and digital application for dentistry without a specific focus, five focused on education and dental school, and two discussed applications in research (see Table 2).

Table 2. Retrieved papers. EHR, electronic health record; mHealth, mobile health; CBCT, con-beam computed tomography; ICT, internet and communication technologies.

Author, Year, Country	Design	Participants	Technology Discussed	Field of Application	Ethical Issues
Boden (2008), USA	Theoretical		Digital transfer of patient records	Dental practice	Justice and autonomy- high charges for the patient prevent beneficial use of records for future patient treatment
Calberson et al. (2008), Belgium	Theoretical		Digital radiography	General	Fraudulent use of radiographs
Cederberg and Valenza (2012), USA	Theoretical		EHR (in dental schools)	Dental school	Justice, patient privacy and security, shift in doctor patient relationship, misconduct from students
Chambers (2012), USA	Theoretical		Digital Communication	Dental practice	Shift in doctor patient relationship, patient privacy and security, professionalism
Cvrker (2018), USA	Theoretical		mHealth	General	Patient access, data ownership, patient privacy and security, bystanders
da Costa et al. (2012), Brazil	Theoretical		Teleorthodontics	General	Patient privacy and security
Day et al. (2018), UK	Feasibility Study	Birth cohort in the United Kingdom	Data linkage	Research	Anonymization, data ownership
Eng et al. (2012), USA	Theoretical		Personalized dentistry	General	Discrimination, confidentiality
Gross et al. (2019), Germany	Theoretical		Digitalization in dentistry	General	Shift in doctor patient relationship, data literacy, responsibility and accountability for AI, digital footprint
Indu et al. (2015), India	Empirical	A sample of postgraduate students and teaching faculties of oral pathology in India	Digital photography	General	Anonymity and security
Jampani et al (2011), India	Theoretical		Teledentistry	General	Confidentiality, patient privacy and security, consent
Kapoor (2015), India	Empirical		Digital photography and radiology	General	Fraudulent use of radiographs/photographs, scientific misconduct
Khelemsky (2011), USA	Theoretical		CBCT	Dental practice	Harm to patient, consent
Knott (2013), UK	Theoretical		ICT	Dental practice	Anonymity, data security, patient privacy
Luther (2010), UK	Theoretical		Digital forensics	Research	Fraudulent use of images, scientific misconduct,
Neville and Waylen (2015), UK	Theoretical		Social Media	Dental practice	Shift in doctor patient relationship, patient Confidentiality, privacy, anonymity
Oakley and Spallek (2012), USA	Theoretical		Social Media	Dental School	Shift in doctor patient relationship, patient privacy and confidentiality, miscommunication, boundary violation
Peltier and Curley (2013), USA	Theoretical		Social Media	Dental practice	Dishonest/unlawful advertising, patient confidentiality
Rao et al. (2010), India	Empirical	A sample of randomly selected clinicians in India	Digital photography	General	Fraudulent use of photographs, scientific misconduct
Spallek er al. (2015), USA	Theoretical		Social Media	Dental School	Shift in doctor patient relationship, patient privacy and confidentiality, miscommunication, boundary violation
Stieber et al. (2015), USA	Theoretical		Electronic media and digital photography	Dental School	Patient privacy and confidentiality, autonomy and consent
Swirsky at al. (2018), USA	Theoretical		Search engine optimization	Dental practice	Beneficence, autonomy, consent, conflict of interest and undue influence

Table 2. *Cont.*

Author, Year, Country	Design	Participants	Technology Discussed	Field of Application	Ethical Issues
Sykes et al (2017), South Africa	Theoretical		Social Media	Dental practice	Patient privacy, anonymity, confidentiality and consent, professionalism, shift in patient doctor relationship, misleading advertisement
Szekely et al. (1996), USA	Theoretical		EHR	Dental practice	Patient privacy and confidentiality, security
Wenworth (2010), USA	Theoretical		Digital Radiography	Dental practice	Patient privacy and confidentiality, misleading advertisement
Zijlstra-Shaw and Stokes (2018), UK	Theoretical		Big Data analytics (in dental education)	Dental school	Consent and data ownership

3.1. Implementation of Digital Technologies in Dentistry

Two papers generally discussed the ethical implications that ICT and digitalization are introducing in dentistry [32,33]. According to Gross et al. [32], digitalization of dentistry is influencing the patient doctor relationship as the integration of digital technologies could distract attention away from the patient during the visit. Issues of data literacy can arise for both the dentist—who will need to constantly be updated on the latest technologies—and the patient—who will need to understand how new technologies work, possibly disfavoring people with poor computer literacy such as the elderly. The application of AI for diagnostic purposes could create issues of responsibility and accountability. A shift might occur towards overtreatment of the patient owing to increased demand for the use of digitized systems. In addition, the constant use, refurbishment, and replacement of increasingly new technology leaves a remarkable digital footprint and aggravates digital pollution. Finally, digital technologies create issues of data security, data falsification, and privacy issues regarding identifiable patient information [33].

3.2. Big Data and Data Analytics

Nine papers discussed the increased employment of Big Data and data analytics in dentistry related to different applications such as data linkage [34], data analytics in dental schools [35], personalized medicine [36], EHRs [37–39], and mHealth and teledentistry [40–42].

3.2.1. Electronic Health Records (EHRs)

Three papers focused on the implementation of EHRs both in private practices and in dental education [37–39]. Ethical issues that arise from this technology are data security, as sensitive patient information could be more easily accessed by unauthorized third parties, resulting in a breach of patient privacy and confidentiality [38,43].

In addition, Cederberg and Valenza [38] argue that the use of digital records might compromise the doctor patient relationship in the future, as easy access to all relevant information through digital means and forced focus on the computer screen could accustom students to becoming more detached from patients.

Suggested solutions for privacy and security issues related to EHR are as follows: (a) the implementation of a three-zone confidentiality model of medical information for databases both linked (networked) and non-linked (network), where different levels of access and security are put in place for different areas—from a more secured inner area that holds the highest sensitive information about the patients (e.g., HIV status and psychiatric care) to an outer, less secured area containing generally publicly available information [37].

3.2.2. mHealth and Teledentistry

Ethical concerns related to mHealth and teledentisry—that is, the use of information technologies and telecommunications to provide remotely dental care, education and raise oral health awareness—were raised by three articles [40–42]. As for other Big Data technologies, issues of data security and patient anonymity [40,41] and confidentiality [42] were the most mentioned, as networked transfer through unsecure means could enable unwarranted third parties to obtain easier access to sensitive patient data.

mHealth might also have an impact on consent both for the patient who might not have been appropriately informed about all of the risks that teledentistry implies [42] and for non-consenting bystanders, whose data might be collected by the device the patient is using [41].

Furthermore, Cvkrel [41] argued that first, mHealth creates additional vulnerability as smartphones gather additional data that are usually not collected by healthcare practitioners (e.g., fitness data, sleep patterns), and, as it is an object of everyday use, it might be easily accessible to unauthorized people. Second, easy access through the smartphone to raw data including data related to dental care could be counterproductive and harmful for patients who might self-adjust the prescription given by the practitioner.

Among the suggested solutions are the following: (a) the establishment of secured networking communication such as the development of state-of-the-art firewalls and antiviruses to mitigate security concerns in telecommunications [40]; (b) the formulation of high quality consent processes that appropriately make the user aware of the risks and all relative factors [41]; and (c) the implementation of information and education about the specific issues that such technology raises for dentists who want to employ teledentistry in their practice.

3.2.3. Personalized Medicine and Data Linkage

In the context of data linkage in dental practices, personalized medicine, and dental schools, the analyzed articles reported how consent issues might arise concerning data usage when the student or the patient cannot be completely informed about the ways in which the collected data is used [35]. Data anonymization [34] and patient confidentiality [36] were again both mentioned as issues of data linkage. Finally, Eng et al. [36] highlighted how discrimination based on higher risk for specific diseases might appear from the linkage of different databases in personalized medicine.

In order to overcome these issues, Eng et al. [36] suggested to develop protective measures at both at a legal and a clinical level to ensure patient data confidentiality and security.

3.3. Digital Communication and Social Media in Dentistry

Seven papers discussed the impact that the employment of digital communication and social media could have upon dental practices and the dentist–patient relationship [44–50].

According to the retrieved studies, one of the main issues is the possibility that commercial values might creep into the management of private practices' websites and official social media pages [44]. For instance, digital media broadcasts might deliver a distorted image of the practice, resulting in misleading or dishonest advertisement of state-of-the-art dental technologies or dental practices, thus exercising an undue influence on patients [47,49]. In addition, Swirsky [50] also raised a concern regarding unethical search engine optimization, an aggressive marketing technique aimed at making your own website appear before others in popular search engines. This practice creates conflict of interest between the dental profession and the patient/public.

Furthermore, the introduction of digital communication in dental practices has heavy effects on the dentist–patient relationship. Neville and Waylen [45] indicate how the use of social media pages is blurring the personal and professional divide. Via social media, patients might have access to information about their dental providers that could compromise the doctor–patient relationship and create issues of trust between the two parties. For instance, shared posts and messages of doctors might be misinterpreted by the users (patients) and be considered unprofessional. Likewise, privacy issues might occur in the case where a dentist visits the personal social media page of their patient and uncovers information that the patient did not want to share with them [46,48]. In addition, doctor–patient confidentiality could be breached by dentists both willingly and inadvertently, if information about a patient is disclosed online, such as identifiable patient photographs or sensitive treatment details [47,49].

Suggested practices to avoid such issues are the development of adequate social media policies for the use of social media in dental practices and increased education for dental practitioners regarding online professionalism in social media—such as awareness of the ethical issues and of the rules of conduct to be used while using social media [48,49].

3.4. Digital Photography and Radiography

The technology discussed by eight of the collected papers was digital photography and digital radiography [51–58]. Among them, four articles [51,53,55,56] highlighted that image modification, made easier by digitalization of both dental photography and radiography, could result in misconduct in science and fraudulent use of modified pictures. Practitioners could be tempted to modify radiographs to deceive insurance companies [51] and researchers might do the same to falsify the results of their research [55].

Three papers correlated the ethical issues of digital imagery to digital sharing and storage of images [52,57,58]. For instance, issues of security of data and patient privacy and confidentiality might arise owing to inattentive storage of images (if digital photographs are stored for too long on an SD-card or if images are shared via electronic means such as using emails and smartphones or networking apps as Whatsapp) [52]. In addition, Stieber et al. [57] indicate how even patient autonomy and consent might be breached if the images are used in an unauthorized manner, such as posting them on a public forum.

Finally, one paper that discussed the ethical issues of digital dental imaging focused on a particular diagnostic technology: cone beam computed tomography (CBCT) [54]. Highlighted issues related to this particular technology are related to its routine use potentially causing harm to patients, especially children and adolescents, owing to the excessive exposure to radiation and consent if patients are not appropriately informed about the health risks they are exposed to when undergoing this diagnostic exam.

Some papers also highlighted some potential solutions. Regarding image modification, the application of state-of-the-art anti-forgery techniques was suggested [51], as well as the development of appropriate guidelines to set an acceptable standard for image modification in dentistry [53]. As for image sharing issues, Stieber et al. [57] suggested the implementation of a privacy compliant framework, where informed consent is enhanced in order to give patients more control over how their images are used, while Indu et al. [52] proposed the use of only custom apps built exclusively for medical data sharing.

3.5. Digital Dentistry Might Solve Ethical Issues

Finally, almost one-third of the papers discussed not only ethical issues, but also mentioned how some of these technologies could be of assistance to solve ethical issues in dentistry and oral health. For instance, the application of digital technologies could result in empowerment of patients and democratization of oral health knowledge owing to increased and widespread information that could be easily retrieved on the Internet [32]. mHealth and teledentistry were argued to be powerful tools to (a) fight known inequalities in healthcare and provide better treatment and patient care in vulnerable populations thanks to the increased saturation of mobile phones and communication technologies that will allow them easier access to health information and remote treatment [41]; (b) overcome cultural and geographic barriers in oral health [40]; and (c) help eliminate the disparities in oral health care between rural and urban communities [42]. Provision of information about health care prevention and oral health issues through social media could positively influence and promote oral healthcare [46,49]. The implementation of research through correlation and data linkage between birth cohorts in the United Kingdom and oral health habits could ameliorate public oral health issues such as caries prevention for children and adolescents [34]. Finally, digital forensics, that is, the digital analysis of images, could help with the recognition of scientific misconduct in dental research [55].

4. Discussion

The analyzed literature raised a plethora of intertwined ethical issues across different technologies and practices in dentistry. Numerous issues are in line with the commonly mentioned ethical challenges that digital technologies are introducing in healthcare—privacy anonymity, security, and so on. On the other hand, additional aspects emerged for dental medicine—such as commercialization and image forgery—that are usually less associated with digitalization of healthcare and Big Data [28].

The most frequently mentioned ethical issues related to the increased digitalization of dentistry are those related to patient privacy, which is often associated with anonymization and confidentiality. This is in line with a study by Mittelstadt and Floridi [28] that highlighted how this cluster of issues related to patient privacy is the one that is most correlated by scholarly research with Big Data technologies such as data analytics, IOT, and social media use. In the era of digitalization, with increased implementation of EHRs and digital data management, issues of privacy become among the most paramount, notably also in dentistry, on account of the opportunities for patient treatment development and research offered by data linkage. Important ethical issues could be overlooked if it is assumed that dental health data are less sensitive than, for example, mental health or stigmatizing infectious disease data. On the contrary, dental health data are sensitive for a number of specific reasons. For example, economic or marketing discrimination, that is, inequality in pricing and offers that are given to costumers based on profiling, such as insurance or housing [59], or discrimination based on health data and health prediction [60], are practices that are creeping out of the exploitation of digital records and might be exacerbated by the analysis of dental records and the use of mHealth in dentistry.

Informed consent was another issue that was often mentioned by the selected papers, although surprisingly not in relationship to the reuse of EHR data. From an ethical and legal point of view, consent needs to be specific concerning three different activities: use for clinical care; clinical trials, where new Big Data technologies are used in dental patients; and secondary use of data for research or other purposes (such as marketing). For use in the clinical setting, issues of informed consent are not so prominent as the EHR would function as a substitute for a paper patient chart, leaving more concerns in the area of data security and patient privacy. However, as Big Data applications for secondary use of EHR data are becoming an increasingly implemented research practice and issues of consent for EHR and Big Data are quite often discussed for the biomedical context [28], more research should be spent in this area for the dental field. In fact, only three retrieved papers focused on EHR—they mostly targeted clinical care, and two of them were from before 2010, which may explain why they did not consider the implications of Big Data and secondary use of data from health records that are currently causing dilemmas of consent from both an ethical and a regulatory point of view [17,61]. Consent was also briefly mentioned by the retrieved papers in relation to data linkage and personalized medicine, but overall, the literature has not sufficiently analyzed the issue data linkage and secondary use of data for dentistry. In fact, electronic dental records increasingly include sensitive and complementary data about the patient, such as automatic tooth charting, general patient health information, development of treatment plans, radiographic captures of the mouth, and intraoral photography [43], which could be linked and analyzed for research and app development purposes without obtaining the appropriate patient's approval. Cvrkel [41], in the context of mHealth, suggested deflecting the discussion from privacy concerns to the development of high-quality consent practices for both clinical as well as secondary research use. On the basis of a recent study by Valenza et al. [62], which assessed the benefits of "Smart consent" strategies that take into account patients' preferences and desires regarding both treatment and the use of their dental data, we argue that the implementation of better consent policies and strategies could also be beneficial to electronic dental records in order to face not only privacy issues related to clinical care, but also issues of consent related to secondary use of data.

As might be expected, considerable space was given to digital photography and radiology in dentistry. Ethical issues were raised in two directions. First, concerns of patient privacy and anonymity and of data security were highlighted in relation to the storage and sharing of digital images [52,57,58]. These issues are of a comparable nature to those enumerated for EHR, mHealth, and teledentistry, which principally have to do with possible access to sensitive patient information by unwarranted parties and interception of digital communications. Interestingly, substantial weight was given to the topic of image forgery. According to the literature, image modification for fraudulent purposes such as insurance fraud and scientific misconduct is described as an expanding practice within dentistry [55,56]. The main problem is that the introduction of digital imagery in our society has exponentially increased the ease with which digital photographs can be manipulated and changed, both in the early and late stages of image production, to a point where essential information about the subject of the image might be falsified [63]. As a consequence, numerous scholars who focused on the epistemic status of photographs and digital imaging have tried to analyze the challenges that digital imaging poses to the epistemic consistency of images [63–65]. The question is, in our opinion, whether in the case of image modification in dentistry, a well-defined line can be settled on acceptable modifications that prevent misinterpretation or misreading by the observer, and modifications that would let the image fall in the category of image forgery. Following clear guidelines on the ethics of image modification [66] could assist practitioners in making the right choices, but might not be enough. Well-intentioned image modification, such as changing the background, modifying light sources, over and under exposure, cropping, color modification, and so on might unintentionally alter the epistemic consistency of an image, as the limit of acceptable alterations that digital images can endure, while maintaining their epistemic value is vague and undetermined [63].

Another interesting finding of this study is that numerous articles—almost one-third of the total and all theoretical papers—rather than expanding on the ethical issues that derive from the application of a medical/dental digital technology, focused on how digital communication could have an impact on the practice of dental care itself and on the doctor–dentist relationship. Some of the retrieved papers [44–49], in fact, highlighted how the inappropriate use of social media by dentists could compromise trust between dental practitioners and patients either owing to leakage of confidential information about patients, such as treatment outcomes or identifiable pictures, or displays of inappropriate behavior on their private social media pages. As the use of social media is permeating our everyday life, blurring the line between private and public, social media and online professionalism are topics that have been increasingly addressed in other areas of healthcare as well [67,68]. The ethical challenge here seems to be twofold. First, education regarding the professional use of social media for dental practitioners could be enhanced by the implementation of rules and social media policies that clearly state the "dos-and-don'ts" of managing a social media page, such as the following: do not post identifiable pictures of patients without their consent; do not discuss patient treatment on the page, and so on [48]. However, if a breach of confidentiality should occur through inattentiveness, the reach of the leaked information would be greater than in face to face exchanges, expanding exponentially the scale of the mistake [67]. Second, it becomes more challenging to implement strategies to appropriately educate dental practitioners about their private social media behavior. It has been argued by Greysen et al. [67] that some online content that might be flagged as unprofessional—such as posts concerning off-duty drinking and intoxication or the advertisement of radical political ideals that might question their professionalism—do not clearly violate any existing principle of medical professionalism, as they are done in the private sphere. In addition, even the interactions that a health practitioner might have with the private social media page of a patient become an intricate matter that might raise ethical dilemmas. By only accessing the page of their patient, the doctor could access private information such as their marital status, sexual orientation, or political orientation that might have an impact, either conscious or unconscious, on the practitioner's personal perception of the patient [69]. Things become even more complicated if the healthcare professional retrieves posts or photos on social media sites that depict patients participating in risk-taking or health-averse behaviors [67]. All of this information might create a fracture in the patient–doctor relationship, as implicit bias and conflict of interests might prevent medical practitioners from providing the patient with the best care [69,70].

In addition, another interesting challenge raised by almost all of the papers that discussed digital communication in dentistry was the issues of commercialization and conflict of interest that interfere with patient care. A strong focus of some of the papers was on the possible exertion of undue influence on the patient by producing misleading advertisement for private practices and state-of-the-art dental procedures. As Chambers et al. [44] argue, the dentist–patient relationship should never shift to one of customer–provider, and commercial interests should always be in a subordinate position to that of oral health, as the well-being of the patient should always come first. In addition, according to the American Dentist Associations' (ADA) Code of Conduct: "dentists who, in the regular conduct of their practices, engage in or employ auxiliaries in the marketing or sale of products or procedures to their patients must take care not to exploit the trust inherent in the dentist–patient relationship for their own financial gain [. . .] and no dentist shall advertise or solicit patients in any form of communication in a manner that is false or misleading in any material respect" [71].

Doing so would negate the patient's right to self-determination and accurate information [50]. As additional technological developments are being increasingly introduced in dental practices, it is of the utmost importance that strong measures are taken to limit commercial interests for dental practice.

In addition, while a substantial number of papers focused on digital photography and radiography, as well as the impact of digital communication for dental practice, this systematic review highlighted some gaps regarding some of the applications that data technologies have in dentistry and the possible ethical issues that might emerge as a consequence. For instance, the implementation of AI applications for diagnostic purposes in dentistry [12] or the sophistication of 3D imaging technologies for pre-operative clinical assessment [9] were not discussed in the retrieved literature. In addition, very few of the retrieved papers focused on the increased application of Big Data analytics and data linkage of health-related data. Shetty et al. [72] highlighted how the debate on digital dentistry is reflective of the traditional dental delivery model and usually focuses on micro trends in technology development such as technology-assisted services (e.g. computer-aided design/computer-aided manufacturing (CAD/CAM)), digital radiography, and electronic patient records. However, trends in the implementations of Big Data technologies such as mHealth, social media, AI, and the like are transforming oral healthcare through social and technical influences from outside the dental profession, as has been seen in relation to the social media use by dental providers. In addition, it has recently been argued that current literature on the topic of digital dentistry has a tendency to focus on its beneficial potentials or on the technical challenges of the discussed technology without appropriately addressing the ethical issues that these technologies might raise [32]. Also, our review indicates that, while a theoretical discussion on this topic is emerging, empirical studies on the ethical issues of digital implementations in dentistry are largely lacking. As a consequence, owing to the sensitive nature of data included in electronic dental records, the specific digital implementations in dental practice and research, and the gaps in the literature regarding the ethical analysis of some dental applications, it is of the outmost importance to conduct additional research, and especially more evidence-based studies, on the possible specific ethical issues related to the field of digital dentistry in order to appropriately understand and confront these issues.

Finally, only a few papers mentioned ethical issues that could be solved by digital dentistry. In addition to those mentioned in Section 3.5, there are two other contenders for useful applications of Big Data research. It has historically been very difficult to conduct epidemiological research on the relationship (if any) between the public health measure of adding fluoride to water supplies and the incidence of dental fluorosis in children owing to the very high number of variables and confounders involved in such research. Big Data analytics could make sense of this difficult area of research, helping to address the public health ethics of water fluoridation [73]. Similarly, antibiotic prophylaxis before dental treatment in patients who have undergone heart surgery remains a contentious area, with dentists tending to recommend against it despite heart surgeons supporting the prescription of antibiotics [74]. Big Data research could help to shed some light on this difficult ethical dilemma.

5. Conclusions

Our study highlighted how most of the issues presented for digital dental technologies such as electronic dental records, mHealth, and teledentistry, as well as developments in personalized medicine, are in line with those mostly discussed in the debate regarding the application of ICT in healthcare, namely, patient privacy, confidentiality and anonymity, data security, and informed consent. In addition to those issues, image forgery aimed at scientific misconduct and insurance fraud was frequently reported in the literature. Moreover, the present review identified how major concerns in the field of dentistry are related to the impact that an improper use of ICT could have on the dental practice and the doctor–patient relationship. In this context, issues of online professionalism were raised together with issues of aggressive or misleading social media or web. Finally, additional research should be conducted to properly assess the ethical issues that might emerge from the routine applications of increasingly novel technologies.

Author Contributions: Conceptualization, M.F., E.D.C., and D.S.; methodology, M.F. and E.D.C.; data analysis, M.F. and E.D.C.; writing—original draft preparation, M.F.; writing—review and editing, D.S., E.D.C., T.J., and B.S.E.; supervision, B.S.E.; funding acquisition, B.S.E. All authors have read and agreed to the published version of the manuscript.

Funding: The funding for this research paper was provided by the Swiss National Science Foundation in the framework of the National Research Program "Big Data", NRP 75 (Grant-No: 407540_167211).

Acknowledgments: The first author would like to thank Christophe Schneble for his support during data collection and analysis.

Conflicts of Interest: The authors declare no conflict of interest. The funders had no role in the design of the study; in the collection, analyses, or interpretation of data; in the writing of the manuscript; or in the decision to publish the results.

References

1. Lynch, C. How do your data grow? *Nature* **2008**, *455*, 28–29. [CrossRef]
2. Boyd, D.; Crawford, K. CRITICAL QUESTIONS FOR BIG DATA. *Info. Commun. Soc.* **2012**, *15*, 662–679. [CrossRef]
3. Mertz, L. Saving Lives and Money with Smarter Hospitals: Streaming analytics, other new tech help to balance costs and benefits. *IEEE Pulse* **2014**, *5*, 33–36. [CrossRef] [PubMed]
4. Cohen, I.G.; Amarasingham, R.; Shah, A.; Xie, B.; Lo, B. The Legal And Ethical Concerns That Arise From Using Complex Predictive Analytics In Health Care. *Heal. Aff.* **2014**, *33*, 1139–1147. [CrossRef] [PubMed]
5. Lee, C.H.; Yoon, H.-J. Medical big data: promise and challenges. *Kidney Res. Clin. Pr.* **2017**, *36*, 3–11. [CrossRef]
6. Liu, X.; Faes, L.; Kale, A.U.; Wagner, S.K.; Fu, D.J.; Bruynseels, A.; Mahendiran, T.; Moraes, G.; Shamdas, M.; Kern, C.; et al. A comparison of deep learning performance against health-care professionals in detecting diseases from medical imaging: a systematic review and meta-analysis. *Lancet Digit. Heal.* **2019**, *1*, e271–e297. [CrossRef]
7. Nilsen, W.J.; Kumar, S.; Shar, A.; Varoquiers, C.; Wiley, T.; Riley, W.T.; Pavel, M.; Atienza, A.A. Advancing the Science of mHealth. *J. Heal. Commun.* **2012**, *17*, 5–10. [CrossRef]
8. Fasbinder, D.J. Digital dentistry: innovation for restorative treatment. *Compend. Contin. Educ. Dent.* **2010**, *31*, 2–11.
9. Joda, T.; Wolfart, S.; Reich, S.; Zitzmann, N.U. Virtual Dental Patient: How Long Until It's Here? *Curr. Oral Heal. Rep.* **2018**, *5*, 116–120. [CrossRef]
10. Finkelstein, J.; Ba, F.Z.; Bs, S.A.L.; Cappelli, D. Using big data to promote precision oral health in the context of a learning healthcare system. *J. Public Heal. Dent.* **2020**, *80*, S43–S58. [CrossRef]

11. Joda, T.; Waltimo, T.; Pauli-Magnus, C.; Probst-Hensch, N.; Zitzmann, N.U. Population-Based Linkage of Big Data in Dental Research. *Int. J. Environ. Res. Public Heal.* **2018**, *15*, 2357. [CrossRef] [PubMed]
12. Joda, T.; Waltimo, T.; Probst-Hensch, N.; Pauli-Magnus, C.; Zitzmann, N.U. Health Data in Dentistry: An Attempt to Master the Digital Challenge. *Public Heal. Genom.* **2019**, *22*, 1–7. [CrossRef] [PubMed]
13. Hogan, R.; Goodwin, M.; Boothman, N.; Iafolla, T.; Pretty, I.A. Further opportunities for digital imaging in dental epidemiology. *J. Dent.* **2018**, *74*, S2–S9. [CrossRef] [PubMed]
14. Vandenberghe, B. The digital patient – Imaging science in dentistry. *J. Dent.* **2018**, *74*, S21–S26. [CrossRef]
15. Brodt, E.D.; Skelly, A.C.; Dettori, J.R.; Hashimoto, R.E. Administrative Database Studies: Goldmine or Goose Chase? *Evid Based Spine Care J.* **2014**, *5*, 74–76. [CrossRef]
16. Liang, H.; Tsui, B.Y.; Ni, H.; Valentim, C.C.S.; Baxter, S.L.; Liu, G.; Cai, W.; Kermany, D.S.; Sun, X.; Chen, J.; et al. Evaluation and accurate diagnoses of pediatric diseases using artificial intelligence. *Nat. Med.* **2019**, *25*, 433–438. [CrossRef]
17. Ioannidis, J.P. Informed consent, big data, and the oxymoron of research that is not research. *Am. J. Bioeth.* **2013**, *13*, 40–42. [CrossRef]
18. Martani, A.; Geneviève, L.D.; Pauli-Magnus, C.; McLennan, S.; Elger, B.S. Regulating the Secondary Use of Data for Research: Arguments Against Genetic Exceptionalism. *Front. Genet.* **2019**, *10*, 1254. [CrossRef]
19. Francis, J.G.; Francis, L.P. Privacy, Confidentiality, and Justice. *J. Soc. Philos.* **2014**, *45*, 408–431. [CrossRef]
20. Schneble, C.O.; Elger, B.S.; Shaw, D. The Cambridge Analytica affair and Internet-mediated research. *EMBO Rep.* **2018**, *19*, e46579. [CrossRef]
21. Schneble, C.O.; Elger, B.S.; Shaw, D. Google's Project Nightingale highlights the necessity of data science ethics review. *EMBO Mol. Med.* **2020**, *12*(3), e12053. [CrossRef] [PubMed]
22. McMahon, A.; Buyx, A.; Prainsack, B. Big Data Governance Needs More Collective Responsibility: The Role of Harm Mitigation in the Governance of Data Use in Medicine and Beyond. *Med Law Rev.* **2019**, *28*, 155–182. [CrossRef] [PubMed]
23. Choudhury, S.; Fishman, J.R.; McGowan, M.L.; Juengst, E. Big data, open science and the brain: lessons learned from genomics. *Front. Hum. Neurosci.* **2014**, *8*, 239. [CrossRef] [PubMed]
24. Favaretto, M.; De Clercq, E.; Elger, B.S. Big Data and discrimination: perils, promises and solutions. A systematic review. *J. Big Data* **2019**, *6*, 12. [CrossRef]
25. Geneviève, L.D.; Martani, A.; Shaw, D.M.; Elger, B.S.; Wangmo, T. Structural racism in precision medicine: leaving no one behind. *BMC Med Ethic* **2020**, *21*, 1–13. [CrossRef]
26. Martani, A.; Shaw, D.; Elger, B.S. Stay fit or get bit - ethical issues in sharing health data with insurers' apps. *Swiss Med Wkly.* **2019**, *149*, w20089. [CrossRef]
27. Martin, K.E.M. Ethical Implications and Accountability of Algorithms. *SSRN Electron. J.* **2018**, *160*, 835–850. [CrossRef]
28. Mittelstadt, B.D.; Floridi, L. The ethics of big data: current and foreseeable issues in biomedical contexts. *Sci. Eng. Ethics* **2016**, *22*, 303–341. [CrossRef]
29. Esfandiari, S.; Feine, J. Health technology assessment in oral health. *Int. J. Oral Maxillofac. Implant.* **2011**, *26*, 93–100.
30. Moher, D.; Shamseer, L.; Clarke, M.; Ghersi, D.; Liberati, A.; Petticrew, M.; Shekelle, P.G.; Stewart, L.A. Preferred reporting items for systematic review and meta-analysis protocols (PRISMA-P) 2015 statement. *Syst. Rev.* **2015**, *4*, 1. [CrossRef]
31. Rodgers, M.; Sowden, A.; Petticrew, M.; Arai, L.; Roberts, H.M.; Britten, N.; Popay, J. Testing Methodological Guidance on the Conduct of Narrative Synthesis in Systematic Reviews. *Evaluation* **2009**, *15*, 49–73. [CrossRef]
32. Gross, D.; Gross, K.; Wilhelmy, S. Digitalization in dentistry: ethical challenges and implications. *Quintessence Int.* **2019**, *50*, 830–838. [PubMed]
33. Knott, N.J. The use of information and communication technology (ICT) in dentistry. *Br. Dent. J.* **2013**, *214*, 151–153. [CrossRef] [PubMed]
34. Day, P.F.; Petherick, E.; Godson, J.; Owen, J.; Douglas, G. A feasibility study to explore the governance processes required for linkage between dental epidemiological, and birth cohort, data in the UK. *Community Dent. Health* **2018**, *35*, 228–234.
35. Zijlstra-Shaw, S.; Stokes, C.W. Learning analytics and dental education; choices and challenges. *Eur. J. Dent. Educ.* **2018**, *22*, e658–e660. [CrossRef]

36. Eng, G.; Chen, A.; Vess, T.; Ginsburg, G.S. Genome technologies and personalized dental medicine. *Oral Dis.* **2011**, *18*, 223–235. [CrossRef]
37. Boden, D.F. What Guidance Is There for Ethical Records Transfer and Fee Charges? *J. Am. Dent. Assoc.* **2008**, *139*, 197–198. [CrossRef]
38. A Cederberg, R.; A Valenza, J. Ethics and the electronic health record in dental school clinics. *J. Dent. Educ.* **2012**, *76*, 584–589.
39. Szekely, D.G.; Milam, S.; A Khademi, J. Legal issues of the electronic dental record: Security and confidentiality. *J. Dent. Educ.* **1996**, *60*, 19–23.
40. Da Costa, A.L.P.; Silva, A.A.; Pereira, C.B. Tele-orthodontics: Tool aid to clinical practice and continuing education. *Dental Press J. Orthod. Rev.* **2012**, *16*, 15–21.
41. Cvrkel, T. The ethics of mHealth: Moving forward. *J. Dent.* **2018**, *74*, S15–S20. [CrossRef] [PubMed]
42. Nutalapati, R.; Boyapati, R.; Jampani, N.D.; Dontula, B.S.K. Applications of teledentistry: A literature review and update. *J. Int. Soc. Prev. Community Dent.* **2011**, *1*, 37–44. [CrossRef]
43. Cederberg, R.; Walji, M.; Valenza, J. *Electronic Health Records in Dentistry: Clinical Challenges and Ethical Issues*; Springer Science and Business Media LLC: Cham, Switzerland, 2014; pp. 1–12.
44. Chambers, D.W. Position paper on digital communication in dentistry. *J. Am. Coll. Dent.* **2012**, *79*, 19–30. [PubMed]
45. Neville, P.; Waylen, A.E. Social media and dentistry: some reflections on e-professionalism. *Br. Dent. J.* **2015**, *218*, 475–478. [CrossRef] [PubMed]
46. Oakley, M.; Spallek, H. Social media in dental education: a call for research and action. *J. Dent. Educ.* **2012**, *76*, 279–287. [PubMed]
47. Peltier, B.; Curley, A. The ethics of social media in dental practice: Ethical tools and professional responses. *J. Calif. Dent. Assoc.* **2013**, *41*, 507–513. [PubMed]
48. Spallek, H.; Turner, S.P.; Donate-Bartfield, E.; Chambers, D.; McAndrew, M.; Zarkowski, P.; Karimbux, N. Social Media in the Dental School Environment, Part A: Benefits, Challenges, and Recommendations for Use. *J. Dent. Educ.* **2015**, *79*, 1140–1152.
49. Sykes, L.M.; Harryparsad, A.; Evans, W.G.; Gani, F. Social Media and Dentistry: Part 8: Ethical, legal, and professional concerns with the use of internet sites by health care professionals. *SADJ* **2017**, *72*, 132–136.
50. Swirsky, E.S.; Michaels, C.; Stuefen, S.; Halasz, M. Hanging the digital shingle. *J. Am. Dent. Assoc.* **2018**, *149*, 81–85. [CrossRef]
51. Calberson, F.L.; Hommez, G.M.; De Moor, R.J. Fraudulent Use of Digital Radiography: Methods to Detect and Protect Digital Radiographs. *J. Endod.* **2008**, *34*, 530–536. [CrossRef]
52. Indu, M.; Sunil, S.; Rathy, R.; Binu, M. Imaging and image management: A survey on current outlook and awareness in pathology practice. *J. Oral Maxillofac. Pathol.* **2015**, *19*, 153–157. [CrossRef] [PubMed]
53. Kapoor, P. Photo-editing in Orthodontics: How Much is Too Much? *Int. J. Orthod.* **2015**, *26*, 17–23.
54. Khelemsky, R. The ethics of routine use of advanced diagnostic technology. *J. Am. Coll. Dent.* **2011**, *78*, 35–39. [PubMed]
55. Luther, F. Scientific Misconduct. *J. Dent. Res.* **2010**, *89*, 1364–1367. [CrossRef]
56. Rao, S.; Singh, N.; Kumar, R.; Thomas, A. More than meets the eye: Digital fraud in dentistry. *J. Indian Soc. Pedod. Prev. Dent.* **2010**, *28*, 241. [CrossRef]
57. Stieber, J.C.; Nelson, T.M.; E Huebner, C. Considerations for use of dental photography and electronic media in dental education and clinical practice. *J. Dent. Educ.* **2015**, *79*, 432–438.
58. Wentworth, R.B. What ethical responsibilities do I have with regard to radiographs for my patients? *J. Am. Dent. Assoc.* **2010**, *141*, 718–720. [CrossRef]
59. Peppet, S.R. Regulating the internet of things: first steps toward managing discrimination, privacy, security and consent. *Tex. L. Rev.* **2014**, *93*, 85.
60. Hoffman, S. Employing e-health: the impact of electronic health records on the workplace. *Kan. JL Pub. Pol'y* **2009**, *19*, 409.
61. Starkbaum, J.; Felt, U. Negotiating the reuse of health-data: Research, Big Data, and the European General Data Protection Regulation. *Big Data Soc.* **2019**, *6*, 2053951719862594. [CrossRef]
62. Valenza, J.A.; Taylor, D.; Walji, M.F.; Johnson, C.W. Assessing the benefit of a personalized EHR-generated informed consent in a dental school setting. *J. Dent. Educ.* **2014**, *78*, 1182–1193. [PubMed]
63. Benovsky, J. The Limits of Photography. *Int. J. Philos. Stud.* **2014**, *22*, 716–733. [CrossRef]

64. Hopkins, R. Factive Pictorial Experience: What's Special about Photographs? *Nous* **2010**, *46*, 709–731. [CrossRef]
65. Alcarez, A.L. Epistemic function and ontology of analog and digital images. *CA* **2015**, *13*, 11.
66. Cromey, D. Avoiding twisted pixels: ethical guidelines for the appropriate use and manipulation of scientific digital images. *Sci. Eng. Ethic* **2010**, *16*, 639–667. [CrossRef]
67. Greysen, R.; Kind, T.; Chretien, K.C. Online Professionalism and the Mirror of Social Media. *J. Gen. Intern. Med.* **2010**, *25*, 1227–1229. [CrossRef]
68. Ventola, C.L. Social Media and Health Care Professionals: Benefits, Risks, and Best Practices. *J. Formul. Manag.* **2014**, *39*, 491–520.
69. Fitzgerald, C.; Hurst, S. Implicit bias in healthcare professionals: A systematic review. *BMC Med. Ethics* **2017**, *18*, 19. [CrossRef]
70. Garrison, N.O.; Ibañez, G.E. Attitudes of Health Care Providers toward LGBT Patients: The Need for Cultural Sensitivity Training. *Am. J. Public Heal.* **2016**, *106*, 570. [CrossRef]
71. McCarley, D.H. ADA Principles of Ethics and Code of Professional Conduct. *Tex. Dent. J.* **2011**, *128*, 728–732.
72. Shetty, V.; Yamamoto, J.; Yale, K. Re-architecting oral healthcare for the 21st century. *J. Dent.* **2018**, *74*, S10–S14. [CrossRef] [PubMed]
73. Shaw, D.M. Weeping and wailing and gnashing of teeth: The legal fiction of water fluoridation. *Med Law Int.* **2012**, *12*, 11–27. [CrossRef]
74. Shaw, D.; Conway, D. Pascal's Wager, infective endocarditis and the "no-lose" philosophy in medicine. *Heart* **2009**, *96*, 15–18. [CrossRef] [PubMed]

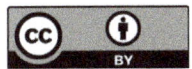

© 2020 by the authors. Licensee MDPI, Basel, Switzerland. This article is an open access article distributed under the terms and conditions of the Creative Commons Attribution (CC BY) license (http://creativecommons.org/licenses/by/4.0/).

MDPI
St. Alban-Anlage 66
4052 Basel
Switzerland
Tel. +41 61 683 77 34
Fax +41 61 302 89 18
www.mdpi.com

International Journal of Environmental Research and Public Health Editorial Office
E-mail: ijerph@mdpi.com
www.mdpi.com/journal/ijerph

www.ingramcontent.com/pod-product-compliance
Lightning Source LLC
LaVergne TN
LVHW070547100526
838202LV00012B/407